Information Processing in Motor Skills

Ronald G. Marteniuk
University of Waterloo

wcb
Wm. C. Brown Publishers
Dubuque, Iowa

BF
455
.M337
1976

To Vi plus Kim, Lisa and Jason

Copyright © 1976 by Holt, Rinehart and Winston

Copyright © 1989 by Wm. C. Brown Publishers. All rights reserved

Library of Congress Catalog Card Number: 75-43982

ISBN 0-697-06292-9

No part of this publication may be reproduced, stored in a retrieval system, or transmitted, in any form or by any means, electronic, mechanical, photocopying, recording, or otherwise, without the prior written permission of the publisher.

Printed in the United States of America by Wm. C. Brown Publishers
2460 Kerper Boulevard, Dubuque, IA 52001

10 9 8 7 6 5 4 3 2

Preface

Increased interest in motor skill acquisition has produced voluminous amounts of literature in the form of research papers and books. However, in the main these works have approached skill acquisition in a piecemeal fashion, leaving the prospective teacher or researcher in a quandary when he attempts to synthesize the countless facts arising from this literature. As Gentile (1972) states:

> The area of motor skills seemed to have a supermarket quality: a little massed/distributed practice here, feedback there, stacks of reaction time, mental rehearsal, speed/accuracy, short-term memory, and other distinct topics of interest piled about in disarray.

If a synthesis of this material is attempted, what usually results is a set of principles that are either so general as to be completely unusable or, at the other extreme, are applicable to only very specific conditions. Regardless of the outcome, what results is a set of principles that are incapable either of contributing to a basic understanding of motor skill acquisition or of assisting an individual in making decisions regarding the applied problems faced in teaching motor skills. Perhaps Adams (1971) has best summarized the reason for this state of affairs:

> The villain that has robbed "skills" of its precision is applied research that investigates an activity to solve a particular problem, like kicking a football,

flying an airplane, or operating a lathe. This accusation sounds more damaging than intended, because applied research is necessary when basic science lacks the answers. Nevertheless, the overall outcome of applied research is a collection of answers on specific problems, practically important to someone at a particular moment but not the steady building of scientific knowledge that can some day have power to answer all the problems. Instead of asking about variables, laws, and theories as scientists do, investigators of skills have asked about tasks and efficiency in them as engineers do. The latter is important and necessary but no substitute for the former.

With this in mind, this book is an attempt to present the student who wishes to study motor skills with an overall, basic view of the processes that underlie man's ability to perform and learn motor skills. The presentation is based on the belief that a student, whether he be a potential teacher or researcher of motor skills, must have a unified concept of how man performs and learns skills.

Before we proceed to the task at hand, however, a word of caution is appropriate. The area of motor performance and learning is a complex topic and any book, out of necessity, runs the risk of presenting an oversimplified view of the processes involved. It must be realized, therefore, that not only are the views expressed in this book just one specific approach to the topic but that also, since knowledge is continually being gained in this area, this approach will continually need updating and modification. Nevertheless, the philosophy behind this book is that one must start from a conceptual state and work toward the concrete world. Without a theoretical perspective on how individuals perform and learn skills, a student cannot generate the ideas needed to solve practical problems or to bridge the existing state of knowledge with the yet undiscovered aspects of human motor behavior. Thus, rather than being a book on "what to do" when a specific situation arises, it is hoped that the knowledge the reader gains can be used to help bridge the gap between what is now known and what needs to be known in the future.

Finally, one last delimitation seems to be necessary before proceeding to the content of this book. The approach to be taken in studying information processing in human motor performance and learning is basically one delimited to the behavioral level. A major objective of this book, based on observation of human behavior in well-controlled settings, is to infer from this behavior what central nervous system mechanisms underlie or subserve this behavior. It is true that another valid approach to studying the same type of behavior would be from a physiological viewpoint, where the neural events underlying behavior become the main interest. This latter approach, however, is beyond the scope of this book. There is no doubt that the motor behavior discussed in the following chapters depends upon the activity of the brain and that the fields of physiology and biochemistry have made large advances in understanding these activities. However, at the same time these fields of inquiry do not necessarily answer the questions that are of most vital concern to the individual studying motor behavior. Neisser (1967) perhaps best described the contrast between the study of brain process from behavioral versus physiology-biochemistry perspectives when he gave the analogy between man and computer. He stated that the task of understanding human behavior from a behavioral perspective is analogous:

... to that of a man trying to discover how a computer has been programmed. In particular, if the program seems to store and reuse information, he would like to know by what "routines" or "procedures" this is done. Given this purpose, he will not care much whether his particular computer stores information in magnetic cores or in thin films; he wants to understand the program not the "hardware." By the same token, it would not help the psychologist to know that memory is carried by RNA as opposed to some other medium. He wants to understand its utilization, not its incarnation. (Neisser, 1967, p. 6).

In essence, then, the purpose of this book is to study how individuals use information and not how this information is physiologically or biochemically stored. There is no doubt that some of the knowledge from these fields will at times help the student of motor learning better understand motor performance and learning, but these approaches are, for the most part, beyond the scope of the present book.

R. M.

Waterloo, Ontario
January 1976

Contents

Preface   iii

Section 1
INTRODUCTION TO THE HUMAN PERFORMANCE MODEL   1

Chapter 1
The Human Performance Model and Definition of Terms   3

    INTRODUCTION   3
    THE HUMAN PERFORMANCE MODEL   5
        The model defined   5
        Human performance theory and the limiting principle   6
        Memory and the human performance model   8
    DEFINITION OF TERMS   12
        Information   12
        Information processing   12
        Information transmission   12
        Perceptual-motor skill   13
        Perceptual-motor performance vs. learning   13
        Feedback   13
        Proprioceptive and kinesthetic feedback   13
        Knowledge of performance (KP)   14
        Knowledge of results (KR)   14

Coding of information	14
Plan of action	14
Motor commands	15
Movement execution and control	15
Open and closed skills	15

Chapter 2
The Human Performance Model Applied to an Analysis of Perceptional-Motor Skills and Teaching — 17

OPEN SKILLS	18
The perceptual mechanism	19
The decision mechanism	23
The effector mechanism	24
CLOSED SKILLS	27
The perceptual mechanism	27
The decision mechanism	28
The effector mechanism	28
COMMUNICATION (TEACHING)	29
Two components of communication skills	30
Perceptual mechanism	31
Decision mechanism	33
Effector mechanism	33
SUMMARY	33

Section 2
THE EXPANDED HUMAN PERFORMANCE MODEL — 37

Chapter 3
Attention and Human Perceptual-Motor Performance — 39

ATTENTION AS ALERTNESS	39
Determinants of activation	42
Individual differences and activation theory	44
The inverted-U hypothesis explained in information processing terms	45
ATTENTION AND THE LIMITED INFORMATION PROCESSING CONCEPT—A THEME	46
SUMMARY	48
SUGGESTED READINGS	48

Chapter 4
The Perceptual Mechanism — 50

INFORMATION DETECTION	51
Signal detection theory	52
Signal detection theory applied to perceptual-motor skills	58
INFORMATION COMPARISON	61
ABSOLUTE JUDGMENT (RECOGNITION)	64

DETECTION, COMPARISON, AND ABSOLUTE JUDGMENT OF KINESTHETIC INFORMATION	67
Definition of kinesthesis and its sensory receptors	68
Detection of passive movement	69
Active movement	70
Absolute judgment	72
SELECTIVE ATTENTION	75
SHORT-TERM INFORMATION MEMORY	85
Short-term memory defined	85
Capacity of short-term memory	87
Rate of loss of information from short-term memory	90
Interference in motor short-term memory	93
Facilitating retention of information in short-term memory	95
ANTICIPATION IN PERCEPTUAL MOTOR PERFORMANCE	98
Anticipation in hitting or catching a ball	99
Anticipating proprioceptive feedback	100
ANTICIPATION AND TIMING OF MOVEMENTS	101
Effector anticipation	101
Receptor anticipation	101
Perceptual anticipation	102
SUMMARY	102
SUGGESTED READINGS	103

Chapter 5
The Decision Mechanism — 106

REACTION TIME AS A MEASURE OF DECISION TIME	106
MEASUREMENT OF INFORMATION	108
INFORMATION AND DECISION TIMES	111
Temporal uncertainty	111
Event uncertainty (choice reaction time)	112
Perceptual discrimination	115
Practice and compatibility	116
Successively presented signals (the psychological refractory period)	120
TIME AND ATTENTION AS LIMITING FACTORS	123
SUMMARY	126
SUGGESTED READINGS	126

Chapter 6
The Effector Mechanism — 128

FACTORS LIMITING INFORMATION PROCESSING IN THE EFFECTOR MECHANISM	129
Amount of information	129
Attention demands of movement control	135
CONTROL OF "CONTINUOUS" MOVEMENT	138
Levels of movement control	139
Anticipation of feedback	141
Motor programs in the execution of movement	142

HIERARCHICAL ORGANIZATION AND CONTROL OF MOVEMENT	144
Hierarchical and sequential organization	144
Motor programs and the hierarchical control of movement	148
SUMMARY	150
SUGGESTED READINGS	151

Section 3
LEARNING 153

Chapter 7
Information Processing in Perceptual-Motor Learning 155

INTRODUCTION	155
PERFORMANCE MODELS THAT INCORPORATE THE "MOTOR" PERMANENT STORE	157
SHORT-TERM MOTOR MEMORY IN LEARNING	160
THE SCHEMA AS MOTOR MEMORY	168
The development of the schema	169
Intersensory integration and the schema	170
The concept of the motor program redefined	176
KNOWLEDGE OF RESULTS AND PERFORMANCE	177
The role of knowledge of results and knowledge of performance in learning	177
Principles of use of knowledge of results and performance	179
SUMMARY	184
SUGGESTED READINGS	184

Section 4
APPLICATIONS AND IMPLICATIONS 187

Chapter 8
Applications of the Information Processing Model to Motor Performance and Learning Problems 189

INTRODUCTION	189
A TEACHING MODEL	190
Motivation and alertness	192
Formulation of the goals of performance	193
Selective attention	193
Formulation of the plan for action	196
Short-term memory	197
Performance evaluation and feedback	201
THE TEACHING MODEL AND PHASES OF SKILL LEARNING	203
The cognitive phase	205
The associative phase	207
The autonomous phase	211

THE TEACHING MODEL AND OPEN VERSUS CLOSED SKILLS	212
The motor schema of open and closed skills	213
Implications for teaching closed skills	217
Implications for teaching open skills	218
TRANSFER OF LEARNING	221
MENTAL PRACTICE	223
GENERALITY AND SPECIFICITY OF PERCEPTUAL-MOTOR SKILLS	225
Specificity of perceptual-motor skills	226
Specificity of skills and transfer of learning	228
Implications	230
SUGGESTED READINGS	230

Bibliography   **232**

Index   **241**

Section 1

Introduction to the Human Performance Model

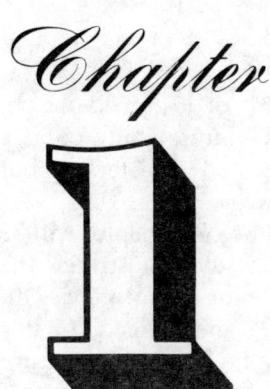

The Human Performance Model and Definition of Terms

Introduction

In the past, books of motor performance and learning have tended to treat this subject as a conglomerate of many unrelated items that supposedly, when brought together between two covers of a book, constituted a systematic approach to the study of how man performs and learns motor skills. As a result, the student of this area has been filled with facts about transfer of training, specificity and generality, motivation, fatigue, memory, and so on, and then in most cases given some ideas about the practical applications of these principles. However, it is the contention here that this piecemeal approach has actually hindered both the development of knowledge in motor performance and learning and the application of this knowledge to problems of concern to the physical education teacher. The main criticism centers around the fact that there has been no effort to study this subject in a systematic, unified way.

An individual's acquisition of an area of knowledge can be facilitated in two ways. First, the subject matter must be introduced in an orderly fashion that ideally begins with general concepts, and then moves toward more specific facts. Second, the content of the subject matter must utilize, whenever possible, the past experience and future interests of the individual so that he can see how the material is related to his interests. These two principles of learning, then, lead to the development of a unified theme, which can be easily handled and serve as a basis for future study or as a framework within which a teacher can make educated decisions about practical problems he faces in a classroom situation.

Within this framework, then, the purpose of the present chapter will be to present a model of human motor performance that illustrates the theoretical underlying components of perceptual-motor performance. In addition, key words and concepts will be introduced and defined. In this chapter and in Chapter 2, discussion of the model is introductory in nature and, as such, is kept rather simple and general to allow the reader to get an overall idea of how the model is used in the study and understanding of perceptual-motor skills. In later chapters, all of the ideas and issues raised in the first two chapters will be discussed in detail and, where possible, documented by research findings. It is expected that the first two introductory chapters will aid the reader in the interpretation and understanding of these more detailed discussions.

Thus, of central concern now will be to identify the underlying information processing mechanisms that contribute to perceptual-motor performance. In this respect the reader should be aware of the fact that the information processing model to be presented is valid only for the analysis of perceptual-motor *performance* in that it can tell us only about the present ability of the performer to process information. Conceivably, a performer could be tested periodically on a given skill and it might be shown that his central nervous system increases in information processing ability because of maturation and increased experience. In this case, however, the information analysis tells us nothing about how the individual increased this ability, just that it actually did increase.

The information processing model to be presented in this chapter is limited in that it will tell us nothing about how a performer learns over time. This limitation serves to illustrate the difference between *human performance theory* and *learning theory*. Treating the performer as an information system composed of component parts can be considered a *performance model* in that it provides knowledge about the *current* state of the performer and his ability to process information. On the other hand, this analysis sheds no light whatsoever on the *mechanisms of learning*; in other words, it provides no understanding of those factors that contribute to the storage of information in memory and that lead to retention of perceptual-motor skills. Thus, a discussion of the learning phenomenon will be delayed now and treated separately in a later section of this book.

The Human Performance Model

The Model Defined

The broad area of human performance theory attempts to study how skilled performers utilize information in perceiving, deciding and organizing an action in relationship to the demands placed on them by the environment.

Figure 1 represents, in schematic form, the basic aspects of an in-

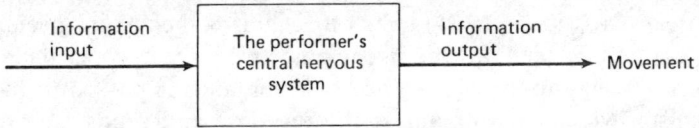

FIGURE 1 A simplified information processing model.

formation processing model. The performer's central nervous system is likened to a communication channel through which information from the environment must be processed. Thus one can conceive of the performer as a communication system, receiving information from the environment (information input) and acting upon it in such a way that what results is a message (information output) that is sent to the muscles so that movement can occur. If the channel or central nervous system has been efficient and accurate in processing the information input, what should result is a movement that is coordinated to the demands of the environment.

To provide a better understanding of the information processing activities of the central nervous system, a more specific human performance model[1] must be used. The one that will be used in this book is one basically

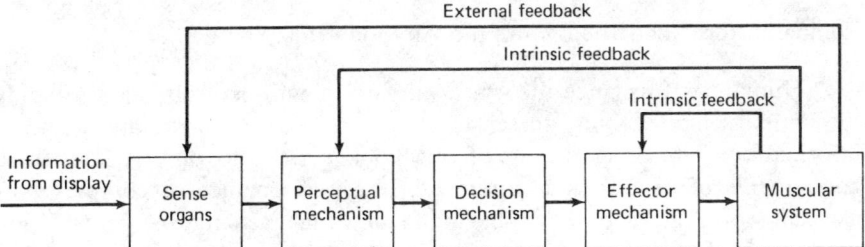

FIGURE 2 The human performance model. From *Readings in Human Performance*, edited by H. T. A. Whiting (Lepus Books, London, 1975) with permission of the publisher.

[1] Human performance theory, a phrase coined by the late Paul Fitts (Fitts and Posner, 1967), is an area of study that attempts to determine man's ability to sense, attend to, store, and transmit information.

similar to that formulated by Welford (1968) and depicted in Figure 2. In essence this model states that there are at least three major mechanisms that mediate information in the environment and movement. The function of the perceptual mechanism, which receives environmental information from the senses, is to provide the central mechanisms with a description of the environment, and it does this by identifying and classifying incoming information. A summary description of the environment in a prearranged code is then sent to the decision mechanism in a sequence of perceptual responses (Crossman, 1964). This mechanism then must decide upon a plan of action in relation to current objectives. Once a particular plan of action has been chosen, a sequence of commands is passed to the effector mechanism, which then organizes the response and sends the appropriate motor commands to the muscular system. Feedback plays an important role in movement execution in that information about the movement can be fed back into the effector mechanism, and allowing, if time permits, corrections to be made as the movement proceeds. The model in Figure 2 also depicts feedback information going back into the perceptual mechanism. Since this feedback loop is longer than the previous one, it would take more time to be processed; but if the movement were long enough, this information could still be used to correct latter parts of the total movement. Moreover, this feedback loop would also provide the performer, after the movement was completed, with information regarding the success of the movement. Questions like "Was the movement performed properly?" and "Did the movement accomplish what was originally intended?" could be answered through evaluation of information contained in this feedback.

Human Performance Theory and the Limiting Principle

Human performance theory, as already mentioned, attempts to study the limits of man's ability to sense, attend to, process, store, and transmit information. The ultimate aim of this book will be to discuss how these components of performance interact in the performance of complex perceptual motor tasks or how they influence the exchange of information between a teacher and his pupils. However since there is little direct physiological evidence concerning how these components or mechanisms operate it is necessary to adopt a "black-box" or behavioral approach to the study of the human performer. What this means is that by careful manipulation of the input information to a performer and observation of his response, inferences are made concerning the mechanisms inside the black box or the central nervous system of the performer. To study only one mechanism at a time, however, is difficult since all three mechanisms, as defined in the human performance model of Figure 2, are within the central nervous system and are undoubtedly simultaneously contributing to any perceptual-motor skill. To overcome this difficulty the "limiting principle" of human performance is utilized; that is, if one is interested in studying only one mechanism, a task is designed whereby successful performance is limited largely by the theoretical mechanisms of interest. The performance of this task then can be used to determine the properties of that particular mechanism. For instance, if one is interested in studying the decision mechanism, a task would have to be designed that did not have significantly large demands on the perceptual and effector processes.

An example of the limiting principle can be derived from analyzing several of the underlying mechanisms involved in being able to hit a pitched ball. Suppose that performance is analyzed according to the model in Figure 2 and, for the sake of clarity at this point, is somewhat oversimplified. From this analysis it is determined that there are three processes involved in hitting a ball: first, the batter's perceptual mechanism must determine what type of pitch (curve, fast ball, and so on) is being thrown and where it will cross the plate; second, the decision mechanism receives this information and then, taking into consideration the present conditions (whether a bunt, sacrifice, or whatever, is required), must decide upon a certain type of swing; finally, the components of the swing must be organized and sent down to the muscles so that the appropriate movements will occur. Now, the overall results could be that the batter misses the ball. From just observing his swing, only one-third (that is, the effector side) of the total performance is noticeable. However, it may be that the pitch was missed because the batter was unable to recognize the type of pitch thrown (the perceptual mechanism) or that the pitch was identified but the wrong course of action was taken by the decision mechanism. Thus performance is seen as being limited in at least three ways, and a breakdown in any one mechanism can lead to poor performance. This leads to an important principle of motor performance: that observing the end result of a motor act is insufficient for determining the reasons for successful or unsuccessful performance.

Now, how does one apply the limiting principle to the above skill so that a more detailed analysis of its component parts can take place? If it is of interest to determine how well baseball players use perceptual cues in a batting skill, one approach would be to place a camera in the batter's box and have a pitcher throw balls over the plate. The film could then be shown to the players and they could be tested as to how fast they can identify a pitch that is going to cross the strike zone or be outside of it; or they might be asked to identify as quickly as possible what type of pitch was thrown.

Of special importance in this "experiment" is the choice of response that the players will be required to use in signaling their answers. Since we are interested in studying the properties of the perceptual mechanism, the limiting principle dictates that the role of the decision and effector mechanisms be kept to a minimum. Thus, the number of alternative motor responses must be kept to a minimum (decision mechanism) and the response must be as simple as possible (effector mechanism). The response that meets both these requirements is a voice reaction time, where the first utterance of a vocal response stops a timer that was started at the beginning of the pitch. This procedure would yield a measure of speed of perception, and the actual words spoken by the player, after the timer has been stopped, would tell whether or not what he perceived was correct.

The underlying assumptions of the above "experiment" is that those batters who have developed the perceptual ability to recognize whether a pitch is a strike or not or what type of pitch is actually thrown should have a faster reaction time than those that lack this ability. If this is indeed the case, the question can then be asked why some players are better than others at this perceptual task. This undoubtedly would lead into a more detailed analysis of perceptual abilities in identifying pitched balls, an analysis that involves examining the various properties or components of the perceptual mechanism. What the prospective teacher, coach, or researcher of ball skills needs, then, is a more detailed description of known properties of the perceptual mechanism so that the resulting knowledge can be applied to his specific interests.

Memory and the Human Performance Model

The model in Figure 2 does not contain an important aspect of human performance—that is, memory. Although the concept of memory is highly complex, it will serve our purpose now to spend some time defining what role this variable plays in motor performance and learning. To be consistent with the organization of this book, memory will be dealt with in both a performance and learning manner. That is to say, some aspects of memory will be important when we study man's ability to process information at a given point in his development, and other aspects of memory will assume importance when the ability to store and retain information is studied.

Posner (1969) perhaps has supplied the most logical breakdown of memory in terms of the purpose of this book. In this article he identifies three types of memory having to deal with the short-term storage of information and, if we add long-term memory to this list, we see that there are four types of memory that are involved, in some way or another, in perceptual-motor skills. For our purposes, we shall label the three types of short-term memory, identified by Posner (1969), as short-term sensory storage, short-term information storage, and short-term operational storage. Although these processes will be dealt with in more detail later, they will be introduced now so that the reader can appreciate where they fit into the general human performance model.

Short-term sensory storage. It has been shown (Sperling, 1960; Keele, 1973) that for a brief visual exposure to several items, there is available for a short period of time (no longer than one second) much more information from that exposure than an individual is capable of recalling. It is as if there is a very short sensory impression of the information from the visual display, and by the time an individual recalls some part of it, the remaining information has faded from this storage system and as a result he is unable to recall it.

In essence this sensory memory system acts like a buffer between initial information input and subsequent information processing activities. This probably adds flexibility to the human's information processing system in that a large amount of environmental information, too much to be all processed, is in a temporary store, and an individual can select items from this store depending upon the unique demands and objectives of current activity.

Thus it would appear that short-term sensory storage is, to a large extent, a function of the peripheral sensory systems that initially transform environmental information to some type of nervous system code. As mentioned above, there is evidence that this type of storage exists in the visual system, and other studies indicate a similar system for acoustical information (Eriksen and Johnson, 1964; Keele, 1973). There is no clear evidence, however, that a system like this exists for kinesthetic or proprioceptive information.

Short-term information storage and long-term memory. Information within the short-term sensory store is either lost very rapidly or it is processed and passed to a second temporary store called short-term information storage. This transfer of information can be thought of as involving a recoding operation that transforms a sensory impression of the information into some code that gives the information a form of representation or meaning that allows it to be retained for at least a short time period and, perhaps, for it to be passed into long-term memory for permanent store. Although there is some controversy over whether short-term memory and long-term memory should be differentiated (Adams, 1967), they can be conceived to lie on a continuum where information enters short-term memory, and if it is rehearsed or practiced, it then passes on to long-term memory.

The time characteristics of short-term information memory are thought to involve the first 20 to 30 seconds after initial presentation of information. After this time, either the information is passed on to long-term memory or else it is forgotten. A second important aspect of this memory system concerns its capacity to hold information. Unlike short-term sensory storage, which appears to have a large initial capacity, short-term information storage is thought to have a relatively small capacity. Thus, not only does it have a short-term interval for storing information but it also can hold only relatively little information, which means that it serves as a bottleneck for the passage of information from the environment to long-term memory.

Operational short-term memory. This last temporary memory is related to short-term information in that it is also concerned with the short-term storage of information. However, unlike short-term information storage, in which information input from the environment is stored, operational memory is more concerned with the storage of information that has been retrieved from long-term memory. The best example of the use of this memory is the case in which an individual is involved in a debate and must form a rebuttal. In order to argue logically, the debater must recall a number of points he wishes to make, logically order them, and then retain both the points for discussion and their sequence while he starts talking and proceeds point by point. It is this temporary storage of information, in a unique combination, that constitutes short-term operational memory. In sports, this memory is also important in that it is probably involved in the formulation of strategies while play is going on. An example would be in tennis where a competitor plans strokes three or four steps in advance which depend not only on how his opponent is playing but also on his ability to recall from long-term memory the best strokes to use against the opponent. He then must retain this strategy for short periods of time while the play unfolds.

The fact that this process is a memory system and subject to loss of information through forgetting is demonstrated by individuals who fail to retain the operations or correct sequence of operations required in a debate or the proper execution of the components of an overall strategy. Often many of us have been left speechless in the middle of presenting our argument because we could not remember the next one or two points, which had been perfectly remembered when we first started.

Long-term memory. Long-term memory is supposedly the permanent retention of information that has been successfully processed by short-term information storage, and through repetitions, rehearsal, or some other process, been transformed into a permanent memory code. Although the code with which verbal and visual information is stored in long-term memory has been investigated to a considerable extent (Keele, 1973), there is an absolute dearth of information on the motor system. It is known that long-term memory for motor skills is very resistant to forgetting, but there is no experimental evidence indicating why this is so. Perhaps once something is known about the form of representation of information in long-term motor memory, some insight will be gained into why motor skills seem to be retained so well over long retention intervals.

Performance versus learning in memory. The above brief descriptions of the different memory systems serve as an overview for future chapters where memory, except for long-term memory, will be treated in more detailed fashion. The purpose of presenting the overview at this time is to attempt to give the reader both insight into the various memory systems and to lay the framework for differentiating between how memory can serve both performance and learning functions.

At the beginning of this chapter a distinction was made between performance and learning, and afterward a human performance model (Figure 2) was presented. To be consistent with this distinction, memory will also be considered both as a performance variable and a learning variable. In later chapters, when learning becomes of major concern, the treatment of the memory of movement will be essentially involved with discovering the way in which information is represented in short-term information storage and the factors that might be responsible for transforming it into a more permanent long-term store. In essence, then, we are interested in how the learner transforms input information in order that it can be retained over long periods of time.

Memory in motor performance, however, is not concerned with the form in which information is stored. Here, the question is more concerned with the capacities of the memory systems (all three short-term systems as previously defined) for retaining information over short time intervals. In other words, we merely ask what limitations memory imposes on the information processing system in terms of how much information can be processed in a given time period. An example would be in determining the number of digits an individual can recall after single presentations of digit lists of varying length. In this case we find the capacity of the short-term information storage system is around seven items (Miller, 1956) and anything more than this capacity will result in errors. Thus this limitation puts an upper boundary on the information processing ability of an individual.

Although performance and learning in memory are not independent, it will be beneficial to treat them so, at least in terms of the performance-learning dichotomy as treated in this book. At times it will be necessary to discuss memory simultaneously from both a performance and learning viewpoint when the distinction, as explained above, is inadequate.

Definition of Terms

The discussion of the human performance model used several terms that must be defined. These definitions not only will aid the reader in understanding this model but also will serve as a basis for the development of future chapters.

Information

Such events as words, movements, and pictures convey information. The more unfamiliar or unpredictable an event is, the more potential information it holds. A demonstration of an overhead clear in badminton would present much more information to an individual seeing this skill for the first time than to an individual who had seen and/or performed it many times before. Thus, amount of information, as used in this context, is directly proportional to the amount of uncertainty an event holds for a given individual.

Information Processing

When an individual performs a perceptual-motor skill, there are a number of central nervous system operations that precede the actual movement. Each of these operations entails the manipulation of information in some way and information processing refers to this use of information leading to movement.

Information Transmission

When an event in the environment contains potential information, and this information is used by an individual to form a movement in response to the environmental information, information has been transmitted. In essence the environmental information acts as an input to the central nervous system operations that precede movement, and the movement acts as the output. The degree to which the output information matches the input information determines the amount of transmitted information. A highly skilled basketball player matches his responses almost perfectly with the game's demands or information and, in this case, most of the input information can be said to be transmitted. The actions of a novice basketball player, however, may only be partially, if at all, correlated with the demands of the game, and hence very little information is transmitted. Thus, to determine the efficiency, as well as the capacity, of an individual transmitting information, the degree of correspondence between input and output information must be determined.

Perceptual-Motor Skill

For the purposes of this book, a perceptual-motor skill refers to those activities involved in moving the body or body parts to accomplish a specified objective. From this viewpoint, movement is seen as only being the end result of a complex chain of information processing activities. Thus the emphasis will be on understanding the information processing activities that precede movement, and for this reason perceptual-motor skill will be treated like a cognitive skill, in which emphasis is placed on the central nervous system's operations that underlie the actual movement.

Perceptual-Motor Performance vs. Learning

Whereas perceptual-motor performance is the current level at which an individual performs a skill, learning is concerned with how he improves this skill. In information processing terms, performance is limited by how much information can be transmitted per unit of time. The study of learning, on the other hand, is more concerned with the form of representation that information in the central nervous system takes. It is assumed that if the way in which information is represented can be understood, considerable insight will be gained concerning how individuals use environmental information to learn a skill. With a knowledge of this process, a teacher might facilitate the learning process by promoting those environmental inputs that are known to be used by the learner in forming a representation of the to-be-learned skill.

Feedback

Feedback is a general, all-inclusive term referring to the information a performer receives about the performance of a skill either while he is performing it or after the skill is completed. Information about feedback is received through any one, or combination, of the sensory systems.

Proprioceptive and Kinesthetic Feedback

Proprioceptive feedback is that information about movement that arises from sensory receptors other than the visual and auditory systems. As such, proprioceptive feedback represents information that arises from a wide variety of sources such as afferent information from the receptors of touch, stretch, pressure, the inner ear (the vestibular apparatus), joints and muscle spindles.

Kinesthetic feedback, on the other hand, though part of proprioception, is defined much more specifically. Usually, kinesthetic feedback is defined (Marteniuk and Hayes, 1975) as movement information arising primarily from the joint afferents and muscle spindle afferents. In some cases the pattern of movement commands, coming from the brain, is also considered to be a part of kinesthesis (Keele, 1968) and is sometimes called efference.

Knowledge of Performance (KP)

KP is the feedback that an individual receives about the actual performance or execution of movement. KP is based upon feedback that is received during the performance of a skill and aids the individual in assessing the correctness of his movements. In terms of the human performance model presented in Figure 2, the implication is that this type of feedback is perceived and stored in memory so that it can be used at a later time for movement evaluation.

Knowledge of Results (KR)

KR is the feedback information that an individual uses to assess whether the objective of the movement was fulfilled. An example would be the visual feedback a basketball player receives as he watches the ball he shot at the basket. By observing how close it came to falling through the hoop he can determine the success of his shot. Successful KR (that is, the ball going through the hoop) is not necessarily related to successful KP (that is, good execution of the movement that propelled the ball toward the hoop) since an individual could perform in far from good form but the ball might still find its way through the hoop.

Coding of Information

Information, whether it resides in the environment or arises from a performer's proprioceptive system, must be transformed into a code that can be used by the performer's central nervous system. All information is first coded physiologically by the receptors into nerve impulses so that this information can be transmitted to the brain. However, in order to be used further, this information must be recoded or transformed into a psychological form that in some way represents the source of the input information. Thus, there are psychological codes for such things as words, pictures, sounds, and information arising from proprioceptive feedback.

Plan of Action

A plan of action, as used in this book, is analogous to an idea or image of a specific movement. Before a specific movement can occur, a plan of action, which specifies the various parameters of the movement, must be formulated. This plan is not only necessary for movement to occur but also is used as a criterion against which the actual movement is compared. In terms of the human performance model in Figure 2, the decision mechanism is responsible for selecting a plan of action that specifies a movement that will suit the needs of the performer in light of specific environmental demands.

Motor Commands

Once a plan of action has been selected, the effector mechanism organizes the necessary motor commands, which will be a sequence or pattern of nervous impulses, and sends these commands down to the muscles to produce the desired movement. One major objective of this book is to study the effector mechanism in an attempt to understand the nature of motor commands. From a human performance viewpoint the question of interest will be to determine the capacity of the effector mechanism to organize and transmit motor commands to the muscles. On the other hand, from a learning perspective the main interest would be to understand how movement information is coded and organized (that is, the internal form of representation movement information takes) within this mechanism.

Movement Execution and Control

Once a pattern of nervous impulses are sent down to the muscles, movement execution occurs. The muscles at this point not only can be considered to be under the control of the initial motor commands but also, after an initial short time lag, be subject to the influence and control of feedback. As will be seen in later chapters of this book, feedback can be used unconsciously or consciously in the execution and control of movement.

Open and Closed Skills

Poulton (1957), in an attempt to define and classify perceptual-motor skills, introduced a concept that has considerable utility for the present book. He classified skills by the type of environment they were performed in. At one end of the continuum were those skills that were performed in environments where the critical cues for the performance of that skill were static or fixed in one position. He called this type of skill a closed skill. Examples of closed skills are gymnastics, bowling, and golf. At the other end of the continuum are those skills that are performed in environments where the conditions under which the skill is performed are continually changing positions in space. These were called open skills, and include activities like basketball, tennis, and football.

When considering these two types of skills in terms of the human performance model presented in Figure 2, it becomes evident that they differentially depend on the three components (perception, decision, and action) of the model. For instance, in the performance of a closed skill, once the skill is begun, interpretation of the environment by the perceptual mechanism would be relatively simple in that the environment is static. However, since environmental conditions are always varying in an open skill, perception of these conditions is of vital importance. Moreover, in open skills the performer must constantly match his output (movement) with environmental conditions, which is no easy task since the conditions are always varying.

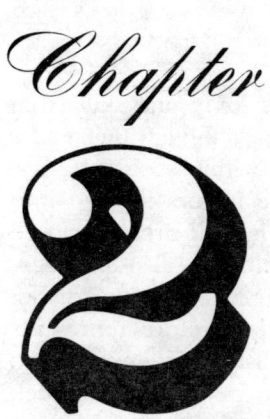

The Human Performance Model Applied to an Analysis of Perceptual-Motor Skills and Teaching

One of the overall purposes of this book is to present the reader with a unified view of human perceptual-motor performance. In Chapter 1 a theoretical model of human performance was introduced. One purpose of the present chapter will be to develop this model further by introducing and defining the various information processes that go into making up the three main mechanisms (perceptual, decision, and effector). This description of the model will be kept simple and introductory in nature so that an overall view can be gained that will facilitate the later detailed analysis (Chapters 3 through 6) of each specific information process within each of the mechanisms.

A second purpose of this chapter will be to demonstrate how the information processing model can be applied to the study and understanding of activities that vary considerably in form. This will be consistent with the view that the information processing model (Figure 2), because it presents a unified view of human perceptual-motor performance, can be used to study almost all perceptual-motor activity, not only from theoretical and research viewpoints but also from an applied viewpoint. Thus, while the various information processes of the human performance model are being introduced and explained, the implications these processes have for the study and understanding of three types of activities will also be discussed. These activities are open skills, closed skills, and teaching. Since there are very many types of open and closed skills, only one skill from each category will be analyzed in terms of the model, although the reader should be able to generalize the analysis to any skill within each category. The open skill used will be a tennis stroke, and the factors that go into successful completion of a stroke will be analyzed. The golf drive, a closed skill, will also be analyzed in a similar manner. Teaching is also analyzed, not only because it is an activity of importance to the physical educator but also because it is really a communication skill and therefore represents another type of information processing activity (as distinct from open and closed skills) that can be described through our human performance model.

The theme of this chapter, then, is that the information processes of the human performance model introduced in Chapter 1 are the underlying mechanisms that produce successful performance in a wide variety of activities. In essence, this means that perception, decision, and action, all central nervous system mechanisms, lie at the base of those activities. It is this very fact that the present chapter will endeavor to illustrate.

Open Skills

One advantage of analyzing an open skill like tennis in terms of the model in Figure 2 is that it emphasizes that performance is composed of several components and that an incorrect response might be caused by any one or a combination of these mechanisms. It may be, for example, that a tennis player may miss a ball he has attempted to hit, not because he is incapable of swinging the racket correctly but because he cannot perceptually identify the characteristics of the ball hit by his opponent. Thus performance breaks down on the perceptual side of our model. On the other hand, just the opposite of the above example might occur in that a tennis player correctly identifies the flight of the ball, knows exactly where it will land and how high it will bounce, and then orders his effector mechanism to organize and initiate an appropriate swing. But this latter process breaks down and as a result the swing does not match the precise characteristics of the ball flight and hence the racket misses the ball.

So far, then, motor performance has produced errors for two entirely different reasons. If we refer to our model again, we can see there is one more mechanism that could cause inappropriate motor performance, and this occurs in the decision mechanism. Conceivably a situation could develop in which an individual could precisely identify the perceptual demands of a skill (perceptual mechanism) and be perfectly capable of organizing and initiating the appropriate response (effector mechanism) to meet the environmental demands. But the existence of these two abilities does not guarantee success since the decision mechanism is an important component of performance and is involved in the selection of the appropriate response, after taking into consideration the current environmental demands and the initial objectives of the performer. It is this decision process, then, that could fail, and the result would be a breakdown in performance. In this regard, performance breakdown might take the form of not being fast enough (this is, the performer took too long to make a decision) or the performer might make the wrong decision.

There is considerable utility in treating motor performance in the above manner in that it serves to emphasize that performance is not only a component process but also the result of an intricate combination of a number of different processes. By studying each process in isolation and then in combination with other processes it is possible to gain a deeper understanding of skilled performance. With this in mind let us now turn to an application of the components of the human performance model to our tennis example.

The Perceptual Mechanism

As mentioned previously, the perceptual mechanism organizes and classifies environmental information and passes this information to the decision mechanism in a series of perceptual responses. This information from the perceptual-mechanism is not only used by the decision mechanism to determine the immediate course of action, but also is stored in memory for use in predictions in later situations. In fact, according to Welford (1958), skilled performance early in the chain of events leading to action depends upon two principles, which can be classified under the term perception: first, that the processes involved in perception are essentially organizing processes; and second, that these processes depend on past actions and experiences.

Our study of the perceptual mechanism, then, will center around attempting to identify those processes that lead to the organization of sensory experience and the influence that past experience has on this process. In addition, the capacity of these processes to transmit information will be studied and inferences will later be made to the operation of the perceptual mechanism in unskilled and highly skilled individuals.

In terms of the role that the perceptual mechanism plays in an open skill consider the example of a tennis player involved in a rally with an opponent. One of the main problems facing the performer consists in reading what his opponent will do and attempting to track the ball in flight once the opponent hits it. Through the use of this information he must then predict where the ball will land and, if it lands in bounds, when and where to initiate a swing to return it.

While the performer is processing this information from the display, he is also receiving another flow of information that also bears directly on his success and is no less important than the display information. This second source of information, derived through vision, audition, and proprioception, concerns not only his position on the court relative to where he will have to be to return the ball properly but also informs him about the position of his limbs (including the current position of the racket) in relation to where they must be to initiate a stroke in order to return the ball.

Finally, a third source of information relevant to the performance of a tennis stroke is the feedback the performer receives both during and after the execution of the stroke. From the beginning of the initiation of the stroke to the contact of the ball the performer may, if time permits, be able to use feedback from his movement (knowledge of performance) to correct any errors in his stroke. In addition, after he hits the ball he may receive feedback from the results of his action (knowledge of results), which will enable him to evaluate the effectivenes of his stroke in terms of what the ball actually did.

In essence then, the performer's perceptual mechanism is more or less bombarded with a large amount of information. What are the information processes within the perceptual mechanism that determine how well he can organize and classify this information? Broadly speaking, these processes can be broken down into three general classes: (1) sensory capacities, which determine an individual's ability to detect, compare, and recognize incoming information; (2) higher-order perceptual processes, which are concerned with information selection and prediction of future events; and (3) memory processes. The combined result of these perceptual processes, in terms of our tennis example, not only should result in a tennis player's knowing exactly what the present situation is in regard to the environment and how his own body is situated within the environment, but also should enable him to predict or anticipate environmental happenings (for example, ball flight) that will occur in the near future.

Since the tennis player is playing in an environment where the cues that govern the play are readily seen, heard, or felt, the limitation imposed by his sensory capacities is probably negligible. In other words, the ability to detect a stimulus, where detection is defined as the least amount of stimulus energy required for experiencing it, and the ability to compare different intensities of the same stimulus, play a small part in sports. The only interest one would have in studying these capacities might be where quantification of the capacity of a certain sensory system (for example, kinesthesis) is desired so as to establish a baseline of information about that system.

However, one sensory process that is of importance to the tennis player, and which has been labeled a sensory capacity, is the ability to recognize information. For instance, the tennis player, when attempting to recognize how fast a ball is approaching him, must compare the observed speed of the ball with a memory for many different speeds. By this process, he is able to place the ball into a category of "fastness." This is not strictly a sensory task since it not only involves sensory information but also requires that this sensory information be compared to past memories of sensory information. This process is called absolute judgment, and as we shall see, it plays a role in many aspects of skilled performance, for not only is it important for recognition of environmental events but it is also involved in recognizing proprioceptive feedback from a movement. In this situation, a player receives proprioceptive feedback from a movement, and before it can be interpreted it must be compared to some memory of past experiences of similar feedback. This comparison results in recognition or classification of the feedback from which further decisions can be made.

Although absolute judgment is a relatively simple process, it is no doubt important for skilled motor performance. Therefore, it becomes of interest to study just how this process limits performance. This can be done, and will be described in a later chapter.

So far we have been discussing relatively simple processes and, as anyone who has played tennis can attest, the game involves much more than this. Perhaps most central to the success of a tennis player is his ability to predict what his opponent will do and to anticipate the flight of the ball as it leaves the opponent's racket. This ability is important because the tennis player is always under the stress of time. Decisions and actions must be made quickly if successful performance is to be achieved. Thus, fast and accurate perceptions of what is happening in the environment must be made.

Anticipation or prediction of future events is a higher-order perceptual process, and is relatively complex. Part of it entails the use of memory, in this case operational short-term memory, where the tennis player has ranked his expectations of what he thinks his opponent will do. In essence he is "looking for" certain things to happen. These expectations, it is argued, influence the tennis player by actually "selectively tuning" his perceptual mechanism to certain aspects of his opponent's movements so that the pertinent information can be gained as quickly as possible (later, this will be called selective attention). If he is correct, a decision about what is happening can be made quickly. However, if his expectations were wrong, he is either caught by surprise or he may be slow in recognizing what is happening; either way the reactions to his opponent's stroke will probably not be very successful.

Although this process is highly dependent on our tennis player's previous experience, there is another way in which predictions about his opponent's actions can be made. This involves the use of the opponent's movements just prior to his contact with the ball and might be termed the recognition of patterns of activity that lead to an expectation of what will happen. It may be, for example, that a highly skilled tennis player is capable of selectively attending to certain of his opponent's actions such that the pattern of these cues leads to an expectation of a certain stroke. In more common words, the opponent is "telegraphing" his actions, a practice that allows our performer to begin to react and move in anticipation of what the opponent will do.

Recognition of patterns of activity, like the previous example of the use of previous expectations, is also highly dependent on memory or past experience. It is almost like a complex absolute judgment in which the sensory aspects of a pattern of movement are compared to a previously stored memory of many different patterns until a match is achieved. This immediately classifies the pattern, and prediction can then be made as to its outcome.

A similar process of pattern recognition might also underlie the prediction of ball flight. If a tennis player is unable to predict, from his opponent's actions, what will happen, his next alternative is to watch the ball, early in its flight path, and attempt to predict its flight characteristics and where it must be intercepted. Since the ball can be traveling very fast, the relevant information must be sensed and recognized early enough to allow time for the tennis player to react and move to intercept the ball. Therefore it is imperative that the tennis player be able to attend to the relevant cues of ball flight so that he can recognize them and successfully make his prediction. Just how much information can be gained about the flight of a very fast ball is, however, open to question. As Scott (1945) has shown, for a fast overhand baseball throw of about 60 feet the batter would have to initiate his swing when the ball was still 20 to 30 feet from the plate in order that the bat would be in position to contact the ball as it crossed the plate. These estimates ignore reaction time, which means that the actual decision to move would have to be made at still an earlier point in time. Since stroked tennis balls can travel just as fast, and faster, than a pitched ball, one can see that in some cases there is not much time to predict ball flight from the ball itself. A good tennis player then, obviously picks up much information from the actions of his opponent and less from the ball once it is stroked.

Although the above processes involved in recognizing or perceiving the environment are important for good tennis, they are not the only sources of information that the perceptual mechanism is concerned with during a rally. As Figure 2 indicates, there is also information coming back to this mechanism in the form of feedback from a player's movements as well as from the consequences of his movements. All this information must be evaluated by the player if he is to complete his movements successfully. In essence, this evaluation of feedback is similar to the problems faced in processing information from the external environment. In fact, in another chapter it will be shown just how the processes of absolute judgment, selective attention, and prediction apply to the perceptual interpretation of feedback information.

The Decision Mechanism

Once our tennis player has correctly recognized or anticipated what type of return his opponent has sent him, the next major process is involved with deciding how to intercept the ball so that it, in turn, can be returned to the opponent. There might also be a decision not to do anything if he believes the ball to be traveling out of bounds. Specifically, however, a course of action must be chosen that will achieve the outcome previously established by the tennis player—that is, to win the rally.

One of the major characteristics of an open skill like tennis is that a large number of possible actions can be taken on each stroke. The action that is finally taken not only must correspond to the specific demands of the approaching ball but also must be made within the framework of how the player wants to return the ball. In other words, the tennis player not only must decide upon what type of stroke he will execute, but also the manner (lob, smash, drive, and so on) in which he wants to stroke the ball and the location in his opponent's court to which he wants it to go. These types of decisions are all relatively dependent on the perceptual information gained from the perceptual mechanism and must be rapidly calculated if success is to occur.

The primary task of the decision mechanism, then, is to decide upon a plan of action by selecting from memory an appropriate plan that will suit the specific needs of the situation. The plan of action is analogous to the performer's idea of what kind of stroke will be necessary to successfully return the ball. As such, a decision must be made as to what kind of stroke will be used (such as forehand, backhand, or overhead) as well as how the general stroke must be modified to meet the exact demands of the approaching ball. It stands to reason then that an experienced tennis player, or for that matter a relatively inexperienced player, will have a large number of plans that he has previously learned and used for tennis and he must now select one of these. As one might expect, this selection takes time and can account for a considerable amount of the total time that is required to process the input information into a response. In fact, if the tennis player had no idea in advance as to what plan of action he might use, the time taken to select the correct one would be considerably longer than the time it would take for his opponent's return to reach him. This implies, then, that a player can prepare himself in advance by bringing the plans he will most likely use from long-term memory to short-term operational memory and in this way reduce the possible number of alternative plans he must eventually search among. In fact, this is probably one characteristic that distinguishes a good tennis player from a novice. The experienced player will prepare alternative courses of action in advance and save considerable time in the search process as compared with the novice, who has no idea what he will do until he perceives the environmental demands.

Another property of the decision mechanism that speeds up the search for the correct plan of action is related to the amount of previous experience in the game and is concerned with the degree of association that a player has developed between specific environmental demands and the specific plans of actions required to match those demands. This is known as stimulus-response compatibility and refers to the ease or rapidity with which a player perceives a particular movement belonging to a specific environmental situation. The more experience one has in a game, the more apparent these relationships become. Thus an inexperienced player, compared to an experienced one, is at a disadvantage in two respects: first, he is unable to prepare in advance the most likely plans of action; and, second, he does not readily associate a given motor pattern with a specific event. Therefore he must "sit and ponder" the situation before coming to a final decision. Both these processes increase the time taken to transform an input into a final action.

In addition to the fact that the above processes serve to limit a tennis player's information processing capacity, there is one more property of the decision mechanism that adds another limitation. This is concerned with the opponent's attempting to deceive (fake) our tennis player into believing a certain type of return will be made, and thereby cause our player to make a decision about what courses of action to take, and then at the last instant executing a different type of stroke. If our tennis player has initiated the decision process (that is, has begun searching for a plan of action appropriate to the fake), he will be unable to make the second decision regarding the actual stroke executed by his opponent. This phenomenon, known as the psychological refractory period, points out the fact that the decision mechanism is capable of making only one decision at a time and cannot make a second one until the first decision has been completed. As suggested above, the fake, which puts the decision mechanism in a refractory state, is effective even if the player does not actually begin to move in response to the fake. All that is necessary is to have him begin the search for an action since he cannot amend this process until the search is completed, by which time the opponent's second course of action has resulted in a return that cannot be acted upon.

The Effector Mechanism

Up to this point in time, our tennis player has perceptually identified what he believes his opponent is doing or going to do, and has decided upon what course of action to take in response to this situation. This plan of action is then used by the effector mechanism to organize the appropriate motor commands and send them down to the muscles. The effector mechanism is thus responsible for selecting and integrating the necessary motor commands that will eventually produce the desired movement.

How is a plan of action (for example, a forehand stroke) organized in the effector mechanism to allow for the efficient execution of movement? To answer this the principles of hierarchical and sequential organization must be explained. A plan of action for a skill like the forehand stroke in tennis, as explained previously, is a performer's broad generalized idea about what is involved in this skill. In order for the plan of action to be carried out, two operations would have to be performed by the effector mechanism. First, the components of the forehand stroke would have to be specified and hierarchically ordered. Hierarchical organization implies an ordering of information from general to specific. Thus the plan of action or the idea of movement would be the most general information, and the various components of the forehand stroke (stance, grip, backswing, and so on) would be more specific information organized within the plan. However, each one of these large components of the stroke can also be subdivided into finer component parts. For instance the stance could be broken down into position of the feet, angle of knee flexion, trunk position, and the like. Thus each one of the broad components would have more specific information organized within them. In essence, then, if one considers the broad plan of action for a forehand stroke as broken down first into relatively broad component parts and then each of these as further broken down into more detail, a hierarchy of information is developed. It is exactly this type of organization that must occur in the effector mechanism for efficient movement to take place. Each one of the component parts of the forehand stroke would have some kind of internal representation that was capable of producing the appropriate motor commands that would in turn produce the desired movement when sent down to the muscles.

Hierarchical organization by itself, however, is insufficient to produce skilled movement. A second type of organization, sequential organization, is also necessary. Without the proper sequence, the components of the skill could be executed in any order resulting in, for example, initiation of the forehand stroke before the correct stance had been obtained. Sequential organization implies that the performer is able to execute the components in the hierarchy in a manner that will produce a sequence of movements logically ordered and designed to meet some specific objective.

Obviously, the level of learning a particular performer has reached greatly influences the degree to which he must consciously organize movement information within the effector mechanism. One would expect that for highly skilled tennis players the lower levels of organization within the hierarchy describing the forehand stroke would be "run off" without any conscious organization. In fact, a major difference between the organization of the effector mechanism of an experienced tennis player and a novice is that the former has a number of "motor programs" at his command. Motor programs, from this point of view, would be highly overlearned plans of actions stored somewhere in the brain and capable of being run off automatically once the performer has ordered their execution. This means that the performer would not consciously have to organize (that is, hierarchically and sequentially organize) each stroke, and thus his burden in terms of processing information would be greatly lessened. The novice, on the other hand, having very few appropriate programs, would consciously have to organize the plans of actions, and thereby greatly add to the complexity of the skill. Although the concept of the motor program is an intuitively appealing explanation to account for highly skilled performance, there are other equally valid explanations. This topic, as well as other topics germane to the development of the effector mechanism, will be discussed in a later chapter.

The last point to be considered under the effector mechanism concerns what our tennis player has to do if he detects an error in the execution of his stroke. Although there are many reasons for an error occurring, two of the major errors would be: (1) Something has gone wrong with the sequential execution of the skill. (2) The stroke has to be modified somewhat as a result of the ball's not following the course of flight that the performer initially predicted. In either of these cases, and for any other case where corrections to current action are required, the use of feedback is implied, where feedback is compared to some reference that enables an ongoing monitoring of the stroke. In the case of sequential mistakes, the performer, by comparing proprioceptive feedback from the stroke to some past memory of what a correct stroke feels like, can detect errors of execution and initiate action to correct the mistake. A similar process of correction might also occur as a result of the tennis player's visually determining that the ball is not going to follow the predicted course of flight.

In both of these cases, the time necessary to make corrections is a vital factor in determining success. If the approaching ball is traveling very fast, a premium is placed on the tennis player's correctly planning everything in advance and correctly executing his plan of action. If the ball is traveling slower, there is time to make corrections. The point is, however, that corrections of movement imply information processing in stages or components similar to those described previously under the perceptual and decision mechanisms of our model. One can now appreciate the complexity of executing a skill and why an inexperienced performer is bombarded with a tremendous amount of information, and therefore why his performance breaks down.

Closed Skills

There are considerable differences between closed and open skills. For one thing, in closed skills, there is not the stress of time involved in perceiving the environment (perceptual mechanism) and deciding (decision mechanism) what plan of action to select that there is in open skills. However, these two mechanisms certainly are involved in processing knowledge of performance during the execution of a closed skill, and in this respect there is not much difference from what occurs in an open skill.

Probably the main point of difference between these two types of skills lies in the effector mechanism. As will be recalled, in an open skill the performer probably never does the same thing twice in exactly the same way, since the demands of the skill are never exactly the same. Yet, in the closed skill, since the environment is relatively constant not only throughout the performance of the skill but also on different occasions of the performance of that skill, the performer's task, once the skill is performed well, is to attempt to duplicate that movement or series of movements time after time. Thus, whereas in an open skill where flexibility and diversification of execution are desirable, a closed skill demands exact replication of a successful movement pattern.

With these differences between open and closed skills in mind, let us now describe the functioning of the three mechanisms in the golf drive, which can be considered one example of a closed skill.

The Perceptual Mechanism

One function of the perceptual mechanism for the golf drive is probably to define the environmental restrictions that might apply to the drive. The recognition of traps, rough, curvature of the fairway, and prevailing weather conditions are all essential to the alignment of the ball and all have to be interpreted in terms of the golfer's past experiences of how well and far he can hit the ball. Since there is a relatively long period of time for this process to occur, the golfer can take pains to see that his recognition of the important environmental restrictions is accurate.

The perceptual mechanism would also be responsible for classifying incoming knowledge of results during execution of the drive and, for classifying both knowledge of results and performance after the drive was completed. In these respects the information processes discussed under the perceptual mechanism for an open skill would apply and thus need not be mentioned here.

The Decision Mechanism

Once the general environmental restrictions have been identified by the perceptual mechanism, an appropriate response must be selected. Unlike the open skill, there are very few alternative actions to select from. It may be that the decision will be to hit a straightaway drive in the normal fashion. But the particular characteristics of the fairway may just as likely demand a deliberate hook, slice, or some other ball placement that is out of the ordinary. Again, since there is no immediate stress of time to make this decision, the golfer can reflect on this decision for some time.

The Effector Mechanism

Whatever the golfer may decide, if he is an accomplished player he will have available in memory a well-organized plan of action that he has used hundreds of time before and will exactly meet the demands of the environment. This plan of action will include all the components of a drive, starting with the grip and the stance and ending with the correct follow-through in the swing. The whole emphasis will be on attempting to duplicate a sequence of actions that has proved successful in the past. In this respect, the organization and execution of the drive is characterized by hierarchical and sequential organization in an identical manner as that described for an open skill.

While it was tempting to describe the operation of the effector mechanism in an open skill as involving a motor program, the tendency to do so in a closed skill is even stronger. Since there are relatively few alternative ways of hitting a golf ball successfully, one might convincingly argue that there is a motor program for each different type of drive. In this way an individual would just have to select the correct program and then let it control the muscles until the swing was accomplished. As evidence for this, one could cite the ability of professional golfers, who are "in the grove," to duplicate their swing exactly, time after time. This view of motor control implies that knowledge of performance is not used to control the execution of the response. That is, a skilled golfer would be able to blank out the conscious control of the swing completely and let the "program" take over. Although this undoubtedly describes what some golfers attempt to do (that is, ignore the execution of the components of the skill and concentrate instead on hitting it down the fairway), this by no means implies that there is a motor program for the drive. As we shall see later, there is a way in which knowledge of performance can be used to guide the execution of a skill while still remaining at a nonconscious level. This view, of course, would argue against the existence of motor programs per se.

Communication (Teaching)

One of the main aims of this book is to demonstrate how a situation involving communication between teacher and student can be treated in a manner similar to a situation involving the performance of a perceptual-motor skill. In this respect it was pointed out that the information processing model in Figure 2 could be used to analyze both situations. Up to this point we have examined the information processing activities of perceptual-motor skills; now we turn to the teaching example.

Before proceeding with a breakdown of the mechanisms within our information processing model it will be beneficial to consider a major difference between the discussion of open and closed skills and the explanation of teaching that will presently follow. This concerns the fact that in the description of the skills, performers with an extensive background of experience were assumed. That is, they had at their disposal long-term memories of perceptual, decision, and effector experiences that aided them in processing information through the central nervous system. However, in the teaching example, the main concern is with the naive or relatively inexperienced performer who has not accumulated this huge reservoir of past experience to draw upon. What this means, from an information processing analysis viewpoint, is that individuals of this type are faced with a great deal more information (that is, uncertainty) than someone with experience. The naive performer has no basis for making absolute judgments or anticipating environmental events. At the same time he has not yet established compatibility between various environmental demands and their proper actions and, further, has had very little practice in organizing and executing plans of actions. All this means that each step in the information processing analysis must involve the reduction of huge amounts of information, and the result is a slow, methodical response, which is just as likely to be inaccurate or inappropriate as it is to be correct.

To overcome this limitation in information processing, the teacher can manipulate the teaching situation in two ways. First, the rate at which information is presented to the naive performer can be slowed down. For instance, the information load can be considerably reduced by presenting new material slowly or by having the performer walk through a skill so that feedback from the environment, as well as from his movements, is received at a slow rate.

The second way of reducing the amount of information that a performer is confronted with is by reducing the number of events in the environment to which he must attend. A wise instructor might reduce the information load on the performer's perceptual mechanism by removing all distracting events and further simplifying the situation by telling the performer what to expect and when to expect it. Similarly, the instructor can map out exactly what kind of action is needed for the correct response (stimulus-response compatibility) and direct the performer's attention to certain aspects of the execution of the sequence of actions. This way the performer knows exactly what to expect and look for, and the information load on his central nervous system is thereby considerably reduced.

One other point should be made clear before describing the various information processes involved in communication between a teacher and student. It will be recalled that in performing an open skill the performer's perceptual mechanism receives information from two sources: from the environment, which is continuously changing, and from the feedback resulting from his actions. To simplify the performer's situation, and hence reduce information load, some teachers will make the environment constant (for example, a tennis instructor throwing balls to his pupil so that the balls bounce the same way time after time) so that the performer has only to attend to the execution of a stroke. However, as was pointed out earlier, this neglects the important aspect of learning how to predict environmental cues and as a result this part of the learning process is hindered. Just what an instructor should do in this case will be discussed in a later chapter. Until then, assume that whenever the information processing characteristics of the perceptual mechanism are discussed both sources of information are taken into consideration.

Two Components of Communication Skills

Teaching, as mentioned previously, is a communication skill that, when considering a perceptual-motor teaching situation, involves two components. First, there is communication between the teacher and students, where the prime objective of the teacher is to inform the students, through instructions and demonstrations, what is involved in the new skill. Since it is imperative that the students understand this information, the teacher should be aware of those factors that affect the perception and retention of this type of information. Thus, the *method* of presentation of new material should be determined by what is known about the ability of human beings to perceive and retain verbal and visual material. This obviously is a function of the perceptual mechanism.

The second component of communication relevant to teaching perceptual-motor skills concerns the *content* of the instructions and demonstrations. The content is different from the method in which material is presented in that content is concerned with those factors that facilitate a student's ability to transform the instructions and demonstrations into movement. Content should be concerned with describing the characteristics of the to-be-learned skill in terms of its perceptual, decision, and effector components. The learner should have enough relevant information about these processes to produce at least a rough approximation of the desired movement.

In essence, the above discussion implies that a teacher must consider two separate but related aspects of the teaching situation in order that successful instruction can occur. First, a teacher must consider the method by which new instructions and demonstrations are presented. The method of presentation can be facilitated by considering the limitations of the perceptual mechanism in receiving this type of information. Second, the instructions and demonstrations to the learner (that is, the content) should be presented in light of what is known about the information processes that contribute to successful performance. Thus, if a teacher has analyzed a new skill in terms of its perceptual, decision, and effector processes, the instructions should contain relevant information about these processes in order that learning will be facilitated.

To illustrate these two components of teaching, the human performance model will now be applied to some of the issues with which a teacher should be concerned.

Perceptual Mechanism

To accentuate the difference between those considerations that a teacher must give toward the method of presenting information as opposed to the content of the information, the discussion of the perceptual mechanism will be given in two sections—one labeled "method" and the other labeled "content."

Method. The primary objective of the teacher is to insure that verbal instructions and visual-verbal demonstrations of skills are perceived and retained by the learner. This applies not only to the initial "lecture" situation, where a new skill is described, but also to any situation in which a teacher gives verbal or visual feedback to a learner concerning his attempt at the new skill. The teacher's first consideration should be that the learner is motivated to learn. Without the necessary motivation or drive, even the best-structured instructions will be wasted in that they will either be ignored or not remembered for any length of time. Although it is sometimes difficult to induce motivation in students (for example, when an unwilling student must take a required physical education class), the teacher must find ways of getting students interested in learning. Chapter 8 will cover this issue in more detail.

Once motivation has been achieved, the next two important considerations involve the limitations imposed on the learner by attention (more specifically, selective attention) and short-term information storage memory. (Both of these processes will be discussed in considerable detail in a later chapter.) As was pointed out previously, because the naive performer has relatively little past experience in the new skill, information overload can easily occur. Thus the instructor must present the minimum amount of information that will enable the individual to identify and recognize the relevant information in a perceptual way. Not only is limited attention a factor, but also short-term information storage must be taken into consideration. Thus, on the one hand, the instructor can describe what the students must attend to in the new skill, but on the other hand if these instructions exceed the short-term memory capacity of the students the information will soon be forgotten. As was discussed previously, the number of events (amount of information) must be reduced if the naive performer is to be successful in retaining the information about the new skill. Memory also plays an important role in instruction because it is limited in terms of the time it can hold information. Hence the instructor must also be aware of the time between presentation of instructions and the first opportunity for students to transform these instructions into an attempted movement. If this interval is too long, some students may forget a substantial part of the initial instructions.

Attention and short-term information storage memory is also important for receiving feedback from the skill during and after its execution. A beginning performer must be able to discern between what he attempted (that is, the teacher's description of the skill) and what he actually did. To do this, memories of *both* these states are necessary. The instructor can facilitate memory of feedback by telling the performer to attend to only certain aspects of the skill as he attempts to perform it. By this is meant that the instructor attempts to simplify the skill in a manner that will allow its execution in a rough approximation of what is required and at the same time keep its information load low enough to allow the retention of its more important features by the performer. In this way the total information load is kept within the capacity of the performer, and he can then make the necessary comparisons between required and actual movements.

Content. To enhance the performance of a new skill, which in turn will facilitate its acquisition, the teacher must include in the description of the new skill those factors that will help the learner perceptually identify the relevant environmental or proprioceptive cues that control the execution of the skill. In closed skills this may not prove to be too difficult, but open skills demand the development of anticipation or prediction of environmental events. Thus careful consideration must be given to what relevant cues the learner is directed to attend.

Decision Mechanism

In closed skills, assuming that the instructor has kept the description of the skill within the perceptual capacity of the performer, there should be no confusion as to what plan of action must be selected to accomplish the skill. However, in an open skill there may be a situation in which one of two alternative plans of action is necessary depending on the specific environmental demand. Here the instructor could spend some time describing the relationship between environment and response so as to enhance compatibility between these two states. This does not really assume great importance when there are only two alternatives because as the performer becomes more capable of performing an open skill there will be a greater number of alternatives available to him and at this point stimulus-response compatibility significantly influences performance. At this level of performance a teacher might be wise to spend considerable time describing the relationships between specific situations in the environment and their appropriate responses.

Effector Mechanism

Even for the most naive performer, except for the very young, there is a considerable amount of sophistication in the organization of the effector mechanism. Although perhaps he has never performed the new skill per se, the performer usually is capable of performing it by utilizing plans of actions already acquired for different purposes. The instructor, in initially describing the skill, should take advantage of this fact by verbally explaining how past motor experience can be transferred to the new skill. An example of this would be a tennis instructor comparing the grip on the racket to a handshake.

Further, since established skills are hierarchically and sequentially organized, the instructor should introduce a new skill in a form that resembles this type of organization. Obviously, to stay within the perceptual capacity of the performer, this description would have to be greatly simplified, but even in this form it might still facilitate performance. In later chapters a framework for presenting skills in this fashion will be developed.

Summary

The purpose of this chapter was twofold: (1) to expand the description of the human performance model presented in Chapter 1; and

(2) to show how the model might be used to understand the underlying processes in open and closed skills as well as in the communication skill of teaching.

In Chapter 1 it was seen that the basic components of the model were perception, decision, and action. Memory was also considered a basic process that had implications for all three components in that memory for perceptual, decision, and effector events was crucial for both performance and learning of perceptual-motor skills. In the present chapter the description of what was included under perception, decision, and action was expanded. Perception, it was explained, consisted of three general classes of processes: (1) sensory capacities; (2) information selection and prediction; and (3) memory. These processes were described and it was explained that they were involved not only in processing environmental information but also in proprioceptive information received as feedback from the execution of a movement.

The decision mechanism was described as being responsible for selecting a plan of action appropriate to the environmental demands a performer is faced with. This process was seen as taking considerable time, but this time could be shortened if a performer, through the use of memory, could prepare alternate plans of actions in advance and if he were easily able to see the relationship between the environmental demand and the appropriate plan of action (stimulus-response compatibility).

Considerations of the effector mechanism basically revolved around the way in which movement information within this mechanism was organized. Plans of actions were seen as being stored in this mechanism in a hierarchical order and, when a particular plan of action was selected to be executed, the effector mechanism was responsible for imposing sequential order on the various components within the plan of action.

A second objective of this chapter was to demonstrate how the human performance model could be used to analyze and understand a wide variety of activities that concern the physical educator. The first type of activity analyzed was open skills, where tennis was taken as one example of this type of skill. It was seen that all three components of the model (perception, decision, and action) were intrinsically involved in successful performance. Closed skills were also shown to rely on these three components, but the perceptual and decision processes were not under the stress of time that usually occurs in the performance of a closed skill. Finally, teaching was analyzed in terms of the human performance model. Two aspects of the teaching process—consideration of methods of information presentation and consideration of information content—were defined and described. The common theme for both these considerations was the fact that a knowledge of the basic components underlying the human performance model was essential for facilitating the instruction process.

The introduction to the human performance model is now complete. The reader should have an overall impression of what is involved in the model and how it can be used to understand perceptual-motor skills and teaching. Chapters 3 through 7 will present a detailed analysis of the human performance model (Chapters 3 through 6) and the processes involved in learning (Chapter 7). Each of the issues raised in Chapters 1 and 2 will be dealt with and the relevant research evidence presented. In addition, the reader will be given sources of readings that can be used to broaden his knowledge in the basic processes involved in perceptual-motor performance and learning. Finally, the last chapter (Chapter 8) will be similar in nature to this chapter in that it will be practically oriented.

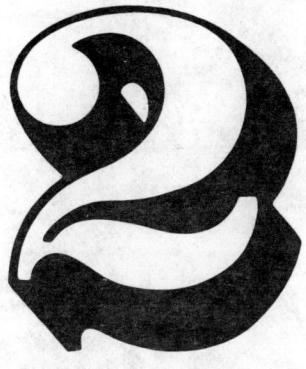

Section 2

The Expanded Human Performance Model

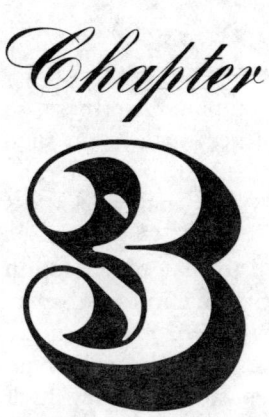

Attention and Human Perceptual-Motor Performance

A concept that will underlie much of the discussion in later chapters of this section is that of attention. Although it is a very nebulous term in that it has many meanings (see Moray, 1970, and Kahneman, 1973, for the various meanings), the concept is important here because three aspects of attention have implications for understanding perceptual-motor performance. These different aspects of attention, described in an article by Posner and Boies (1971), are: (1) alertness; (2) the idea of a limited central processing capacity; and (3) selective attention (the ability to select information of one kind over other kinds). For the sake of organization, only the first two aspects of attention will be discussed in this chapter and selective attention will be treated in Chapter 4, entitled The Perceptual Mechanism, where it more intuitively belongs.

Attention as Alertness

According to Posner and Boies (1971) one aspect of alertness is the ability to sustain attention on a given task over an extended, boring period of time. A related aspect of alertness, more germane to the study of motor skills from the viewpoint of this book, entails the ability to develop and maintain an optimal degree of alertness so that information processing in perceptual-motor performance is maintained at a maximum. Alertness, in this sense, can be thought of as a state of the central nervous system such that it is "ready" to receive and process information at an optimal rate. Any deviation from this optimal state results in a system that works less than maximum.

The above concept of alertness is closely related to that of activation theory where an inverted-U relationship between activation and performance has been postulated. According to Duffy (1962) and, more recently, Birch and Veroff (1966), the activation or arousal level of an individual varies from a very low point during deep sleep to very high levels associated with extreme excitement or anxiety. Arousal is considered to be a neuropsychological concept, referring on the neural side to the state of excitation of the reticular formation of the brain stem, and on the psychological side to constructs such as alertness, attention, tension, and subjective excitement (Fiske and Maddi, 1961).

The importance of activation theory lies in the relationship between arousal and performance. It is hypothesized that for every type of behavior there exists an optimal degree of arousal, usually of moderate intensity, that produces maximum performance. Levels of arousal below or above this optimum amount are seen to produce inferior performance and thus, if one plots performance of a given task over a substantial portion of the arousal continuum, an inverted-U relationship is obtained (Figure 3). This relationship was first postulated by Yerkes and Dodson (1908), and has been dealt with more extensively by Lindsley (1951), Hebb (1955), Malmo (1959), Berlyne (1960), Duffy (1962, 1968), Birch and Veroff (1966), and Scott (1966).

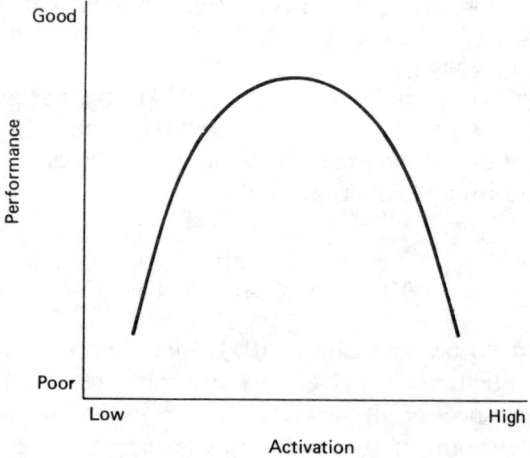

FIGURE 3 Relationship between degree of activation and level of performance.

The relevance of activation theory to the context of this book is the postulation that there is an optimal state of the central nervous system underlying maximum performance. In this respect it is fruitful to conceive of activation as the degree of excitation of the brain stem reticular formation (Scott, 1966) since it is this area of the brain that, upon receiving stimulation, discharges and projects its activity widely into the cortex. Stimulation, as used here, can be thought of as arousing environmental information (a shout, a threat of punishment, a relevant situation), nervous activity caused by receptors within the body (proprioception, pain), or nervous activity from cortical sources (Scott, 1966). Whatever its source, activation theory holds that the reticular formation sends out a diffuse bombardment of nervous activity which effects a generalized cortical arousal, upon which information processing is dependent. As Figure 4 illustrates, the arousal level of an individual influences all aspects of performance. The relevant consideration here, since the teacher or coach has, to some extent, control over the types of sensory stimulation received by his students or athletes, is that it might be possible to regulate these stimuli so that an optimum degree of cortical arousal is maintained. The objective here, then, is to control alertness so that information processing can occur to a maximum extent.

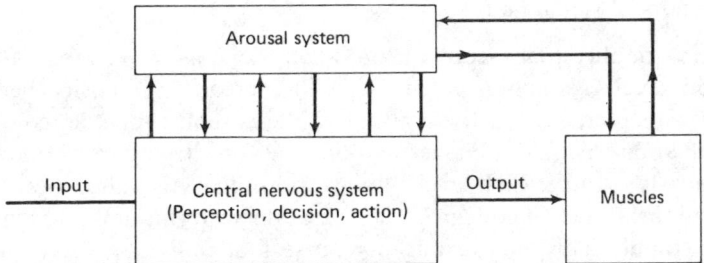

FIGURE 4 The relationships among the arousal system, the muscular system, and the information processing system.

Figure 4 illustrates the relationship between the arousal system as described above and the model of information processing. This figure indicates the interaction among the arousal system, the information processing system, and the muscular system. If one can assume that the brain stem reticular formation is the main arousing system (Scott, 1966), then stimulation from the central nervous system and muscle system activates this system and, in return, nervous activity, which effects an increase in arousal, is sent back to the latter systems.

The model depicted in Figure 4 also implies that there are different classes of stimulation that activate the arousing systems. For one, any increase in muscular tension, which can be thought of as a peripheral source of stimulation, leads to increased arousal. However, stimulation arising from perceptions (for example, seeing a meaningful object), which is a cognitive type of stimulation, could also increase arousal. Hence, the model implies that arousal is dependent not only on physical stimulation but also on higher cognitive activities, such as perception, thinking, deciding, and the like. The model also demonstrates how an inverted-U relationship between arousal and perceptual-motor performance could occur. For instance, it may be that an athlete becomes very stressed upon thinking about an important contest. The model implies that this activity causes an increased arousal level, which is in itself fed back to the central nervous system and muscles. To a point, this increased arousel is beneficial to these systems in that it facilitates information processing and movement, respectively. However, presumably a point is reached where there is too much arousal and either one or a combination of information processing steps breaks down or the muscular system becomes too tense and cannot respond efficiently. Whatever the cause, performance is influenced in a negative manner. In a later section of this chapter, the actual mechanisms of facilitation and impairment will be discussed.

Determinants of Activation

One stimulus that Scott (1966) considers as a variable affecting activation level is stimulus intensity, with increasing intensity being associated with increasing activation level. Here, such things as colors and lights and sounds would all have the potential for varying from a low level of intensity to a rather high level. If activation theory is valid, there should be a relationship between degree of arousal and varying levels of intensity of these stimuli. This is assuming of course that individuals have not become habituated with these stimuli. What this implies is that stimuli that do not vary in intensity can often be ignored by individuals and thus are incapable of producing arousal. For example, a teacher with a monotone voice can easily be "tuned out" by a student, whereas a teacher who varies his voice over a relatively wide range of intensity has more probability of maintaining alert students.

Other variables, perhaps related in some way to the intensity dimension, and postulated by Fiske and Maddi (1961) to increase arousal, are stimulus complexity, uncertainty, meaningfulness, and variation. These are cognitive variables in that they require information processing by the central nervous system before they can influence arousal. These cognitive stimuli would seem to have considerable potential for use by the physical education teacher. By making an experience meaningful to his students a teacher can indirectly influence their attention levels, thus facilitating the instructional process. On the other hand, the judicious use of novel stimuli during instruction can also influence activation level. Finally, making drills or other types of learning situations complex enough to be a challenge, but not unobtainable, is one other way of keeping students alert.

Two other variables that can affect arousal and that seem to be very pertinent to the physical education setting are induced muscular tension and physical exertion. These two variables are related since physical exertion necessarily involves muscular tension but the latter term has usually been used in the context of simple motor acts, such as squeezing a hand dynamometer in one hand while performing a motor task with the other. Other ways in which muscle tension has been induced include such things as hanging weights on the performing arm, pressing springs to the floor with the feet while performing with the hands, or simply holding weights in the nonperforming hand. Much of this work is reviewed by Duffy (1962), Scott (1966), and Marteniuk (1968), and in general they show, though at times not very clearly, that motor performance is facilitated by small amounts of induced muscular tension and inhibited by large amounts. Thus the inverted-U hypothesis is supported, but not overwhelmingly. One reason for the lack of a clear relationship between induced muscular tension and motor performance may result from the methodology used to induce tension. By inducing tension in one limb and performing with another, there is an inevitable division of the subject's attention, which in all likelihood will decrease his performance on the motor task. The larger the tension that has to be induced, the larger the division of attention. The problem is not solved by inducing tension in the performing limb by, for example, attaching weights to the arm that has to track a moving target. In this situation, the total complexity of the motor skill changes as a function of the increasing weight and rather than studying various levels of induced tension (arousal) one ends up studying various levels of task complexity.

The second physical way of varying arousal, that of physical exertion, is currently proving to be a fruitful approach to the study of the effects of arousal on motor performance. Here, arousal is increased through riding a bicycle ergometer or jogging, and results indicate that this arousal not only facilitates motor performance but also increases cognitive skills such as perception and short-term memory. An example of this type of work can be found in a study by Davey (1973), where he had subjects pedal a bicycle ergometer at various work loads. His results indicated that an inverted-U relationship held between work load or level of exertion and performance on a test of mental concentration.

From the above, then, there is evidence to indicate that physical activity, whether static muscular contractions or physical exertion, has an influence on both mental and motor performance, which says in essence that information processing ability is enhanced. These findings obviously not only have implications for instruction during physical education classes, but also can be used to advantage in any situation (regular class room instruction, factory work, desk work) in which sustained attention is required or the possibility of boredom might arise.

Individual Differences and Activation Theory

An additional dimension of activation theory that must be considered when dealing with the inverted-U hypothesis is the inherent level of arousal within different individuals. The inverted-U hypothesis predicts that if an individual is at a low level of arousal, and thus performing less than maximally, his performance can be facilitated by increasing his arousal level. This facilitation of performance continues until an optimum level of arousal is reached, after which any increase in arousal leads to a decrement in performance.

When a teacher or coach is dealing with one individual he may be able to determine just where on the arousal continuum his performer is, and thus increase or decrease stimulation to obtain an optimum level of arousal. However, when dealing with a group of individuals there will probably be individuals whose inherent arousal levels are at all points on the continuum from low arousal to high arousal. That this is so is reflected in the works of personality researchers. For instance, Eysenck (1967) has proposed two personality dimensions that have direct bearing on the inherent arousal level of individuals and how susceptible they are to increases in arousal. The first personality dimension he postulates is a trait called extroversion-introversion and the second one is called neuroticism-stability. Welford (1968) reviews evidence showing how the trait extraversion-introversion is related to the concept of activation and concludes that it is commonly assumed that introverts are by nature more highly aroused than extraverts. Thus, introverts because of their higher arousal level would be expected to perform better on a number of tasks when compared to extraverts.

In terms of the other personality dimension, neuroticism-stability, Welford cites evidence to indicate that neurotic or "unstable" individuals become more easily aroused than stable individuals. From this it follows that an unstable introvert can easily be "pushed over" his optimum level of arousal, which would lead to performance decrement. On the other hand, a stable extravert would conceivably require a relatively large degree of stimulation to reach his optimum level. At any rate, this evidence points to the fact that alertness, as it has been discussed here, is just as much a function of the individual as it is of different types of stimulation.

The Inverted-U Hypothesis Explained in Information Processing Terms

This section on alertness has attempted to show how this variable is linked to the concept of arousal. It has been suggested that alertness, like performance, follows an inverted-U relationship with increasing arousal levels. The question now arises as to what the mechanism of this phenomenon is in terms of the performer's ability to process information. To answer this we must return to the basic information processing model presented in Figure 4. Here the input is processed by the central nervous system, and the resultant is some type of information output. In this regard the central nervous system can be considered a communication channel in which various information processing operations occur. If the channel is efficient, there is a direct correspondence between input and output; but if it is inefficient, the output or the response will not be related to the input.

The task now is to describe how different levels of arousal can retard or facilitate communication through the channel. From this viewpoint, Welford (1968) has formulated a concept that explains the poor operation of the channel at both low and high levels of arousal. He reasons that at low levels the channel is "inert," and the input is lost somewhere in the many information processing steps that are required to transform it into an output. At the other extreme, when activation is too high, this introduces "noise" into the channel so the input is interfered with and confusion arises. Welford reasons that the mechanism behind this noise is the random firing of cortical cells caused by a too intense bombardment of neural activity from the arousal system. The neural activity resulting from these cortical cells being fired masks any input and results in confusion, so high-level judgments or precisely graded responses are impossible to carry out. On the other hand, an optimum level of arousal is seen as sensitizing cortical cells so that they are more readily fired when the appropriate input arrives.

Perhaps this explanation by Welford best illustrates the main point of this section on equating attention and alertness. Such a conceptual framework is valuable in that it outlines a theoretical approach to understanding the process whereby an individual's central nervous system can be aroused or activated in order to prepare it for the acquisition of input information. The relevant points concern the inverted-U relationship between arousal and performance and the fact that for each individual there exists an optimum level of arousal that is associated with maximum performance. However, let it be pointed out that this section on alertness has only attempted to show how an individual can be prepared to receive information. The fact that an individual is optimally aroused and ready to receive information does not necessarily imply that processing of the appropriate information, whether they be instructions from a teacher or cues from a complicated skill, will take place. There are many more factors to consider that limit an individual's ability to process information, with selective attention (to be discussed in the next chapter) chief among them.

Attention and the Limited Information Processing Concept—A Theme

The second aspect of attention, that of a limited central processing capacity, presents a broad view of man as an information processor and, for the purpose of this book, represents a main theme. The idea of a limited central processing capacity comes from the observation that an individual has difficulty in handling two tasks simultaneously. As Keele (1973) points out, if one task cannot be performed simultaneously with another task, then some aspect of both tasks is said to take space. Space in this sense is used to denote the fact that a task requires a portion of the limited processing capacity within the central nervous system. Thus if two tasks both require a portion of this capacity, they interfere with one another and the performance of one or both is influenced adversely.

The above discussion suggests an important principle of human motor performance. That principle arises from equating the processing of information to attention demands or, as Keele (1973) would put it, the concept of space. In essence, this suggests that the processing of information places an attention demand on the mechanisms of the central nervous system. Thus if one mechanism is processing a signal of high information content, this operation requires a considerable portion of the total processing capacity (attention) of the central nervous system, and as a result the operation of the other central nervous system mechanisms may be interfered with. An example of this principle would be to observe an unskilled individual performing a task requiring a relatively complex motor response. Chances are that this act will demand all his attention, and if at the same time he was required to monitor a perceptual display, it would be predicted that he would be unable to perform both at once. An empirical example illustrating this principle is a baby learning to walk. This is a complex effector process for the baby and, as a result, while he is attending to its execution he is oblivious of all environmental information. If he is distracted by something in the environment, such as a loud noise, his attention is switched from walking and in all likelihood he will fall.

This example serves to illustrate the fact that the human being has a limited capacity central nervous system in the sense that information processing requires attention, and once a specific task places an attention demand on some part of the central nervous system other operations are interfered with. The utility of adopting such a conceptual framework can be seen from both practical and theoretical viewpoints. For instance, from a practical viewpoint, a teacher, when presenting to novice performers a skill that requires both complex perceptual and effector processes, should reduce the information load to one of these processes so that the other can be performed successfully. Once one process has been completed successfully a number of times, the second component can then be increased in complexity and both can be performed simultaneously. An example of this would be having badminton beginners practice the overhead clear a number of times in a simulated situation in which the shuttlecock is set up so that they can attend almost exclusively to the execution of the stroke. Once the stroke is completed successfully, the players may then be put into a game situation in which complex perceptual and decision processes must be made concerning the use of the overhead clear.

While later sections of this book dealing with the learning process will discuss to a greater extent the import of the above, it will now be informative to expand the inherent implications that the example has to our information processing model presented in Figure 2. The implication concerns the relationships among the concepts of information load, attention demands, and learning. Inherent in the above badminton example is the concept that when a performer initially undertakes a task, there is usually a great deal of uncertainty in interpreting signals from the display, deciding upon a course of action, and executing the selected motor plan. Each of these three processes places considerable demands on the limited information capacity of the performer. The teacher, by having the performer first practice the overhead clear in a relatively simple situation is, in essence, attempting to reduce the uncertainty or attention demand of the execution of the clear. This is done by allowing the performer to become familiar with the sequence of required actions and the various types of feedback associated with the stroke. Through this practice, uncertainty or information load is decreased, and when the performer enters the game situation he need not attend as much to execution of the skill, thus freeing some of his limited capacity system to cope with the perceptual and decision demands of the game.

By conceptualizing practice as having the effect of reducing uncertainty, which leads to a decrease in the attention demands of the practiced skill, from the viewpoint of information theory and the concept of a limited processing capacity system one can appreciate why a given skill may be complex for one individual but simple for another. Complexity, used this way, is a relative term, and can be equated to attention. If a given skill places a large attention demand on the central processes, it can be considered complex. Walking to a two-year-old baby would be an example of a complex skill in that it requires considerable attention, and if a second task is attempted simultaneously it will interfere with walking. Yet, to the same baby two or three years later, walking is a relatively simple skill, as evidenced by the fact that the child while walking can easily shift his attention to other tasks without hindering the act of walking. The adolescent learning to play a complex game like basketball or badminton proceeds in a similar fashion. At first even the simplest skills involved in a game are attention-demanding, but through practice their uncertainty is reduced—that is, they become redundant—and as a consequence their attention demands are lessened. Through years of practice a skilled individual emerges, and the execution of the various skills are performed without much conscious effort, thus freeing his limited processing capacity to deal with things like the overall strategy of the game.

Summary

In summary of this section, two aspects of the broad area of attention have been presented. The notion of alertness was explained in terms of activation theory. This theory was used to illustrate a mechanism through which an individual's central nervous system is prepared or alerted for receiving information. A second aspect of attention was then presented in which this variable was equated with the concept of limited central processing capacity. From this viewpoint any information processing activity by the central nervous system was seen as causing an attention demand. If two tasks or information processing operations require simultaneous access to this system they compete for the limited capacity and, as a result, interfere with each other. Both of these aspects of attention are important because they not only explain, from a theoretical viewpoint, the processes within the central nervous system that underlie human motor performance, but they also have utility in practical situations where the principles can be applied to teaching and coaching problems.

Suggested Readings

Attention as Alertness

Cofer, C. N., and Appley, M. H., *Motivation: Theory and Research.* New York: Wiley, 1964.

Duffy, E., *Activation and Behavior.* New York: Wiley, 1962.

Martens, R., Arousal and motor performance. In J. A. Wilmore (Ed.), *Exercise and Sport Sciences Review.* New York: Academic Press, 1974.

Posner, Michael I., and Boies, S. J., Components of attention, *Psychological Review*, 1971, **78**, 391–408.

Scott, W. E. Jr., Activation theory and task design, *Organizational Behavior and Human Performance*, 1966, **1**, 3–30.

Attention and the Limited Information Processing Concept

Keele, S. W., *Attention and Human Performance*. Pacific Palisades, Calif.: Goodyear, 1973.

Moray, N., *Listening and Attention*. London: Penguin Press, 1970.

Posner, M. I., and Boies, S. J., Components of attention. *Psychological Review*, 1971, **78,** 391–408.

Posner, M. I., and Keele, S. W., Time and space as measures of mental operations. *Proceedings of the 78th Annual Convention of the American Psychological Association*, 1970.

Chapter 4

The Perceptual Mechanism

As mentioned previously, the perceptual mechanism organizes and classifies input information and passes a series of perceptual responses to the decision mechanism. These perceptual responses are used by the decision mechanism to determine the immediate course of action and also are stored in memory for use in prediction in later situations. Thus the perceptual mechanism is involved in organizing input information and is dependent on past actions and experiences as well. Accordingly, then, our study of the perceptual mechanism will center around attempting to identify those processes that lead to the organization and classification of sensory information and the influence that past experience has on this process.

From an information processing viewpoint the question of interest in studying the perceptual mechanism, and any other information processing mechanism, is how much information it can process per unit of time. In other words, we are attempting to establish the limits of this mechanism to process information. As will be seen, there are several processes within the perceptual mechanism, and each uniquely limits the perceptual process so that only a relatively small amount of input information is actually processed. For example, Crossman (1964) estimates that an individual can remember only about one-hundredth of the information presented in ordinary speech, and thus the perceptual mechanism drastically reduces the information received from the sense organs. A practical outcome of this information reduction arises when one considers the example of an unskilled individual listening to a teacher present a complex description of some motor skill. Usually this individual, if questioned immediately afterward, can accurately remember only a small amount of the total description; the rest is either totally forgotten or reported with great inaccuracy. The challenge to the teacher, in this case, is to realize the limitations that a student has in organizing verbal and visual descriptions and then present material in such a manner that the important points have a good chance of being perceptually organized and retained.

In a similar manner to the problems faced by the teacher, a tennis coach must be aware of his athlete's perceptual limitations when instructing him as to what cues to look for when attempting to read his opponent and the approaching ball. Perception in tennis, as pointed out in Chapter 2, plays a very important role in this game, so the importance of this process cannot be underestimated.

With these examples in mind, we now turn to the processes within the perceptual mechanism that limit information processing.

Information Detection

The first question we ask about the perceptual mechanism concerns the limitations it has in picking up information from either the environment or from feedback, such as proprioception. It has long been known that there are many environmental sights or sounds that are physically measurable but are incapable of being processed by the perceptual mechanism. The study of just how acute the perceptual mechanism is in detecting information is one aspect of a field of investigation known as psychophysics, which is one of the oldest areas of investigation within psychology. Thus, through the use of psychophysics, we can determine just how limited the perceptual mechanism is in detecting information, which is the first process required in information processing if further information analysis is to occur.

The stimulus or lower threshold, which has been used to denote the capacity to detect stimuli, can most easily be thought of as a boundary below which an individual fails to detect a stimulus and above which he always detects it. An example would be to present an individual with a very weak sound. If it was below his lower threshold for sound he would report that he did not hear it. However, if the sound were gradually increased in strength, there would be a point at which the individual would report hearing it. This is the stimulus or lower threshold for that particular sound.

From the name given to the capacity to detect a stimulus (that is, lower threshold), one might expect this to be always the same for any given individual. However, this is not the case. As Woodworth and Schlosberg (1954) report, the best way to demonstrate this is to hold your watch far enough away from your ear so that you can barely hear it. Over a period of one minute you will hear the ticking of the watch become louder and weaker, and in fact at some points you may not hear it at all. This example illustrates the variability of the lower threshold and indicates that our perceptual mechanism has a varying capacity to detect stimuli. Thus, as Figure 5 indicates, rather than there being a fixed stimulus magnitude above which an individual always reports its presence (the dotted line), the actual function is denoted by the solid line. This means that an individual, at times, is capable of detecting stimuli that are usually undetectable and at other times he will not detect stimuli that are relatively strong. Why do individuals exhibit this variability in detection ability? For the answer we turn to signal detection theory.

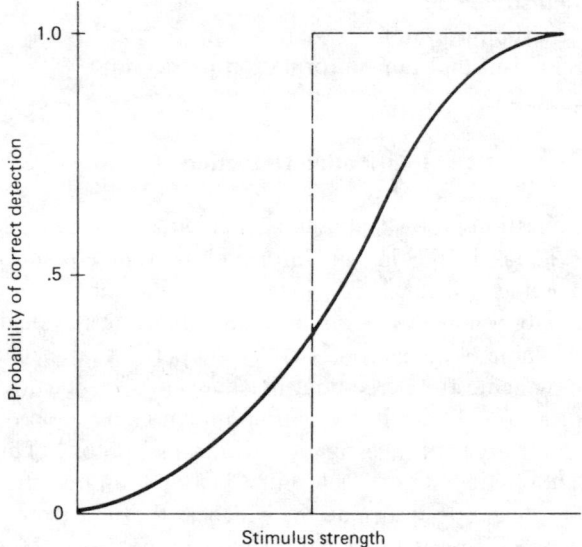

FIGURE 5 Relationship between the intensity of a stimulus and its probability of detection.

Signal Detection Theory

Before we describe the details of signal detection theory, it will be beneficial to develop a theoretical process that supposedly underlies information detection and forms the basis for signal detection theory. In Chapter 3, the topic of alertness was discussed and it was pointed out that the central idea of alertness could be explained in terms of activation theory.

Activation, in turn, was conceived of as a state of nervous activity, within an individual, that varied on a continuum from very low activity (as in deep sleep) to very high activity (as in extreme excitement). In addition, it was postulated that for every individual there is an optimum amount of activation associated with maximum performance for certain tasks. Degrees of activation below and above this optimum amount produced less than maximum performance, but for different reasons.

To explain this decline, the central nervous system of the individual was considered as an information channel through which information was processed. In turn, the success of accurately processing input information was seen as dependent on the state of the channel. At low levels of activation, the neural cells within the channel were seen as being inert and incapable of processing information and as a result information was simply lost somewhere in the channel. At the other extreme, where activation was extreme, the cells within the channel were seen to be overly active and already firing at random. This random neural activity was seen as noise that masked or inhibited the processing of information within the channel and led to a decrease in performance.

The above ideas can now be transferred to the study of the perceptual mechanism. In this case this mechanism can be considered the channel through which input information must be processed. More specifically, for the study of information detection we can conceive of the perceptual mechanism as receiving input information over a relatively large range of different degrees of neural activity. At the one extreme there would be very little neural activity and the perceptual mechanism would be inert and unable to process any information; at the other extreme there would be considerable noise and input information would be confused with this noise.

Let us now proceed with the explanation of signal detection theory. This theory has largely come about within the past ten years, mainly through the work of Swets, Tanner, and their associates (Tanner and Swets, 1954; Swets, 1959, 1964; Swets, Tanner, and Birdsall, 1961; Green and Swets, 1966), and takes as its starting point the fact that the decisions (in this chapter we are concerned with perceptual decisions) an individual makes in real life situations must be made in the face of uncertainty. Uncertainty in perceptual judgments can arise because of the speed of a sensory event (for example, a baseball batter having to identify a baseball, traveling in excess of 100 mph, as a strike or ball) or because the judgment has to be made against a background of noise (for example, a baseball fielder having to find a hit ball with the sun in his eyes).

In signal detection theory terms, any uncertainty that tends to make decisions difficult is called "noise." For example, noise may be inherent in the stimulus that is presented to an individual in that the stimulus might be of poor quality or ambiguous. Or, the noise might occur within the perceptual system itself, which would mask the processing of the stimulus. Noise, in this later example, would be seen as being related to the level of neural activity within the perceptual mechanisms. It is this concept of noise that is directly relevant to our study of signal detection theory because it helps us understand how individuals make perceptual judgments.

When one applies signal detection theory to the study of how individuals make perceptual judgments against a background of noise, caused by random neural activity, two considerations must be made. The first concerns the characteristics of the random neural activity within the individual. For this purpose it is assumed that random neural activity, within an individual, varies over time from a state of relative inertness to one of relatively high activity. However, if one were to plot the amount and frequency of this noise for any given individual observed over a long period of time, one would obtain a function that is depicted in the left curve of Figure 6. This, of course, is a normal curve and indicates that an individual,

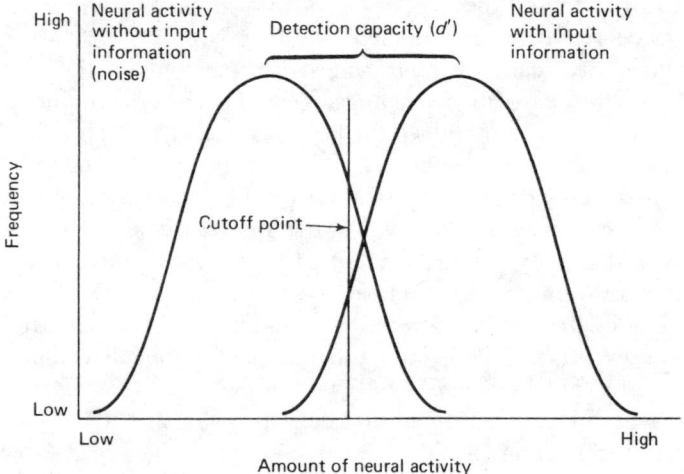

FIGURE 6 Signal detection theory (see text).

over a period of time, will fluctuate from low amounts of neural activity to high amounts, but most of the time he will have an amount of neural activity that is represented by the mean of the distribution. In this case, because it is a normal curve, the mean amount of neural activity occurs at the point on the horizontal axis immediately under the part of the curve represented by the highest frequency. One point to consider, which arises from Chapter 3, is that there would be individual differences in the mean amount of neural activity, possibly as a result of personality differences in the dimensions of introversion-extraversion and neuroticism-stability.

The second important consideration, when applying signal detection theory to how a perceptual judgment is made against this background of neural noise, is the effect that incoming information has on the level of neural activity already present within the individual. In this respect, it is theorized that incoming information causes a constant increase in neural activity that represents a sum of the background, or already existing, activity plus the neural activity caused by the incoming information. Thus, an incoming signal increases the amount of internal neural activity by an amount that is equal to that caused by the signal. Hence, a second distribution, that of neural activity with input information, is created. This distribution is represented in Figure 6 by the right-hand curve.

From a signal detection theory viewpoint, an individual decides whether a signal is present or not by discriminating between the state of neural activity caused by noise alone and the state caused by noise plus the incoming information. If he believes his internal state simply represents random neural activity, his judgment would be that no signal is present. However, if he believes the amount of internal neural activity represents random neural activity caused by incoming information, he would report a signal or stimulus as being present.

As McNichol (1972) points out, the consequences of accepting the concept of decisions being made against a background of internal noise is twofold. First, it reinforces the viewpoint that in human behavior decisions are almost always made in the face of uncertainty, which accounts for the fact that errors in judgment frequently occur. Second, it emphasizes the fact that the internal states of an individual directly influence the way he interprets information from the environment. Factors such as the state of motivation, the past learning experiences, and the attitudes of the individual making the judgment determine not only the efficiency with which he makes judgments, but also tend to bias his judgment towards one type of response rather than another.

The fact remains, then, that an individual must make decisions in the presence of uncertainty. Figure 6 illustrates this by presenting two overlapping distributions of neural activity and the individual's task is to discriminate between them. Because the two distributions overlap, the individual will not always be correct in his decisions. However, signal detection theory proposes that there are two factors that determine the accuracy or inaccuracy with which an individual can make such a decision. The first is the individual's sensory capacity or sensitivity. That is, one can think of an ability, probably neurologically based, that allows some individuals to detect or recognize information at a higher level of sensitivity than other individuals. However, this basic sensory capacity is not the only factor determining an individual's ability to make perceptual judgments. The second factor, which is just as important as sensory capacity, is the degree of bias an individual imposes onto his judgments. Bias, from this viewpoint, can be thought of as arising from the individual's subjective state at the time he is required to make a judgment. Bias thus might stem from an individual's motivational state, from his past experiences in similar circumstances, or from the differential incentives offered him for not making certain types of errors.

An important contribution of signal detection theory is that it allows for the separation of the effects of sensory capacity on perceptual judgments from those effects caused by bias. In this way, this theory is an improvement upon classical psychophysical work, which also attempted to measure sensory capacity. As mentioned at the beginning of this section on Information Detection, this work was characterized by an inability to specify exactly the lower threshold of a stimulus because of the variability of this measure. Signal detection theory would predict that one reason for this variability is the influence that an individual's bias has on his perceptual judgments.

The two parameters of signal detection theory, sensory capacity and bias, are illustrated in Figure 6. Sensory capacity is depicted by d' (pronounced d-prime) and is simply the distance between the means of the two distributions. Bias is reflected in Figure 6 by the vertical line labeled "cutoff point." While it is beyond the scope of this book to explain in detail how these two measures of performance are actually obtained (the reader is referred to the references at the end of this chapter), an intuitive approach to understanding these measures will be presented.

In a typical signal detection experiment, an individual is presented, over many trials and in a random order, one of two types of information. On some trials he is presented with just noise alone and on others he is presented with noise plus a signal. His task on each trial is to report whether or not a signal is present. The simplest example of this situation would be an auditory detection task where an individual must determine whether or not a weak pure tone was or was not present in a burst of white noise.

In this situation, on those trials where just the noise is presented, one can think of this noise adding a constant to the already existing internal background noise caused by the individual's random neural activity. Thus, it would be expected that over many trials where the intensity of the white noise remains unchanged, the amount and frequency of these two sources of noise would produce the normal curve depicted by the left-hand curve of Figure 6. On the other hand, when the signal was embedded in the white noise this would, again over many trials, produce the right-hand curve of Figure 6.

As mentioned before, the individual's task is to discriminate between these two states of neural activity. Signal detection theory holds that the ability to discriminate is partly determined by the sensitivity or sensory capacity of the individual's perceptual process. Practically, sensitivity is seen by the effect that a signal has on the state of neural activity. If an individual has a sensitive perceptual process, an incoming signal will produce larger amounts of neural activity when compared to a relatively insensitive perceptual process. Thus, for those individuals with sensitive perceptual processes one would expect that the right-hand distribution in Figure 6 would be displaced more to the right. In other words, there would be a greater separation of the two distributions and as a result d' (that is, the distance between the means of the distributions) would tend to be large. Conversely, for an insensitive perceptual process the signal would have relatively little influence on the amount of neural activity and d' would tend to be small (that is, the two distributions would overlap to a great extent).

Thus, d' is one way of quantifying an individual's ability to make perceptual decisions. A large d' means that the two distributions in Figure 6 are considerably separated and as a result there is very little uncertainty as to whether or not a signal is present. A small d', however, means large amounts of overlap, and, as a result, an individual would be faced with considerable uncertainty in his decisions. One would expect from this that a small d' would result in a large number of errors.

Notwithstanding the influence that d' can have on signal detection ability, there is still the important influence that the individual's bias has on his accuracy of perception. It is a very rare case where the two distributions depicted in Figure 6 are completely separated which, of course, reflects the fact that in real-life situations, an individual is always confronted with uncertainty in his perceptual judgments. Since this is the case, an individual must set a cutoff point to aid in his discrimination of the two distributions. This cutoff point, depicted in Figure 6, is subjectively set by an individual and, according to signal detection theory, any amount of neural activity that falls below (that is, to the left of) this cutoff point will be evaluated as if it were caused by the neural activity resulting from noise alone. In other words, the individual's judgment would be that no information had been presented. On the other hand, any amount of activity exceeding the cutoff point will be judged as caused by the signal being present. One can immediately appreciate that depending on where the cutoff point is set, certain types of errors will be made.

For instance, a good deal of the time an amount of neural activity that reflects "neural activity with input information" will fall to the left of the cutoff point but will be judged as belonging to the other distribution. Hence the judgment will be that no signal is present, when in actuality it is present. Similarly, there will be occasions when an amount of neural activity reflecting "neural activity without input information" falls to the right of the cutoff point and will be judged as signal present even though no signal has been presented. In signal detection theory terms these two types of errors are called "misses" and "false alarms," respectively.

The placement of the cutoff point, then, has a great influence on the type of errors that an individual will commit when attempting to detect information. If an individual is required to detect a certain type of information correctly and is penalized if he responds that it is there when in actuality it is not, he will shift his cutoff point to the right so that he will give fewer "false alarms." However, notice that the probability of the information occurring without being detected is increased, but, at least, as we have defined that situation, he is not penalized for making this type of error. Conversely, it may happen that it is more important to make correct judgments when a certain type of information is actually present, with false alarms being relatively harmless. If this is the case, the individual will set his cutoff point further to the left to maximize the probability of detecting the information when it is present, but at the same time this increases the probability of false alarms.

While the above description of signal detection theory has been brief, the reader should now have an understanding of the role that both sensory capacity and bias play in perceptual decisions. It should be emphasized again that these two parameters are independent of one another and that signal detection theory offers several ways in which both can be relatively easily quantified. Thus, one could measure differences between people, or groups of people, in terms of both these parameters. Ways in which these measures can be used in the study of perceptual-motor skill will now be discussed.

Signal Detection Theory Applied to Perceptual-Motor Skills

What is the importance of signal detection theory for the study of perceptual-motor skills? Certainly, it is not useful for describing how individuals detect weak signals, since almost all relevant information in perceptual-motor skills and games are well above the minimum level of intensity to be detected. However, the execution of many skills involves processing signals from the environment that are only momentarily present because of the speed with which such things as an opponent, a teammate, or a ball moves. It is in these situations that a performer must make a decision whether a certain cue was present or not, and the accuracy of this decision will affect the eventual outcome of his movement in response to the environment. For example, a basketball player coming down the court with the ball must make quick decisions on what to do with the ball. He must make these decisions in terms of interpreting information he receives from his guard, his opponents as a team, and his teammates as a team. In many cases an environmental situation that demands a certain move or pass to be made will be present only for an instant and, if it is not detected, the opportunity for the player to make the correct move will be lost.

Although signal detection theory has potentially many contributions to make to the study of perceptual-motor skills, only two will be illustrated here. The first use concerns determining the ways in which highly skilled open-skill performers make such rapid decisions regarding the state of the environment they are performing in. According to signal detection theory, there are two reasons the performers can make these fast decisions. One is that their sensory systems may be very acute and as such they detect information in the environment that an average player would not be able to perceive. In other words, referring to Figure 6, their detection capacity or d' is superior. On the other hand, according to signal detection theory, a second reason for their superior ability may be that through experience they acquire some kind of perceptual strategy that leads to increased confidence in making such judgments and, as a result, they set their cutoff point (as in Figure 6) differently than an average player would. Thus, through the use of signal detection theory, a differentiation between the roles that basic sensory acuity and experience play in detecting environmental situations is possible. Since relatively little is known about how highly skilled athletes make decisions, research in this direction would be most valuable.

A second contribution signal detection theory can make to the study of perceptual-motor skills lies in using it to study what happens to judgments about information received while a performer is under stress. Stress, here, is used in activation theory terms, where it is seen as a stimulus that produces arousal. Thus physical fatigue and extreme excitement are classed as stress where both produce arousal levels over the optimum level. Both these variables are frequently found in the performance of perceptual-motor skills. Extreme excitement can be caused by an individual's becoming overly motivated to do well or by the excitement produced by a challenging situation. Whatever the cause, the effect is the same—an increase in arousal.

One researcher who has devoted much time to the investigation of the effects of stress on signal detection ability is Welford (1968, 1973). He has reviewed a large amount of literature in which it is indicated that stress seems to cause an individual to shift the cutoff point in Figure 6 to the left, thus causing more false alarms in the detection of information. This intuitively would seem to describe the overaroused performer who, in the stress of competition (he may be fatigued and/or overexcited), does something totally unrelated to the demands of the situation. It is as if he had expected something to happen, and because his cutoff point is more to the left, he detects that indeed his expectations were correct, but instead his judgment is a false alarm. However, before he can correct his judgment he has carried out the motor behavior appropriate to his incorrect expectations, thus causing a glaring error.

Welford (1973) goes on to describe a more general relationship between arousal and signal detection theory that also has applications to perceptual-motor performance. In essence, his views tie in nicely with the concept of alertness presented in Chapter 3. Welford argues with the fact that stress causes individuals to shift the cutoff point to the left. Instead, he presents a more explanatory theory of what happens under stress by combining activation theory with signal detection theory.

Figure 7 presents three different pairs of distributions, similar to the distributions presented in Figure 6, and each pair with the same cutoff point. One major postulation that Welford makes is that increases in arousal increase the readiness of the brain cells to fire until they are overaroused, at which point they actually fire. This result is reflected in the two distributions (that is, neural activity without input information and

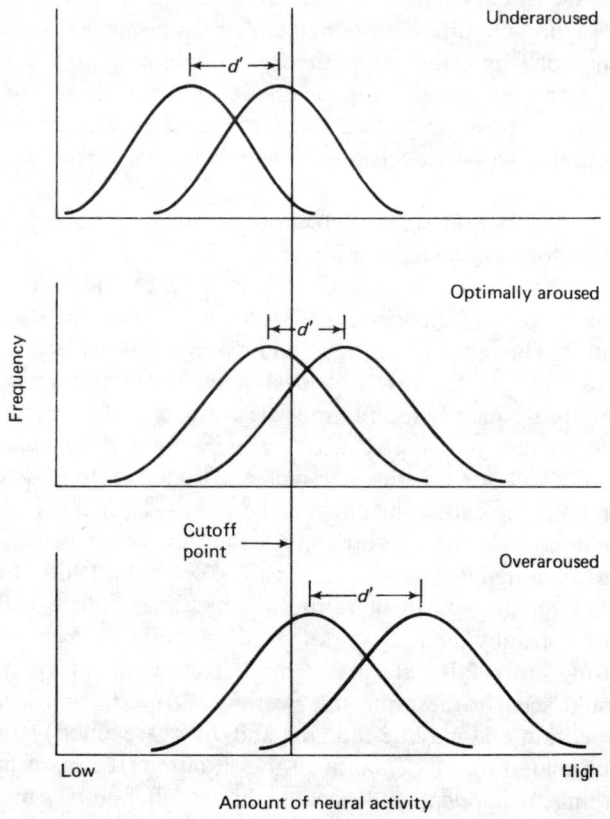

FIGURE 7 Relationship between level of arousal and signal detection ability.

neural activity with input information), increasing in variability but with the ratio between the standard deviations and the distance between their means remaining unchanged.

If the above theory is correct, as can be seen from Figure 7 the underaroused individual, because his central nervous system is relatively inert, makes errors mainly of omission (that is, misses) since on many occasions when the information is present he reports that it is not there. At the other extreme, when an individual is overaroused, he makes errors largely characterized by commission or, in other words, he reports the information present when it is not (that is, false alarms). However, when he is optimally aroused, even though he still makes errors, the number of correct judgments will be in the majority.

Welford's theory would seem to have some applicability to understanding errors in perceptual-motor performance that are attributable to information processing within the perceptual mechanism. Although there is very little evidence to back up the theory, it is intuitively appealing and certainly needs to be considered both in an applied sense as well as for research purposes.

Information Comparison

The preceding section, on information detection, was concerned with discussing factors associated with detecting either low intensities of information or information only briefly present in the environment. Information comparison, in contrast, deals with intensities of information that are present for a considerable time and above the lower threshold, and asks the question of how well an individual can distinguish between different intensities of information from the same information source. An example of the procedure to investigate this ability would be to present to an individual a standard stimulus—such as a light of given intensity. A second light (the comparison or test stimulus), which is of a different intensity, is then presented, and the individual being tested must judge whether the comparison is the same as or different from the standard. Although there are various methods by which the standard and comparison stimuli can be presented (Woodworth and Schlosberg, 1954) the basic aim is to establish a difference threshold or just noticeable difference (jnd), which is a basic measure of a sense's capacity and is defined as the least increase in information intensity required to be correctly reported 50 percent of the time (Woodworth and Schlosberg, 1954).

Does this type of sensory capacity have important implications for studying perceptual-motor skills? To the extent that it involves comparison between different intensities of the same type of information and that an individual is allowed to take as much time as he wants in giving his judgment, it probably has very little to do with the actual performance and learning of perceptual-motor skills. Usually, there is no standard information present with which to compare the "test" information and, moreover, as Fitts and Posner (1967) point out, perceptual-motor skills are usually performed under the stress of time and thus accuracy of judgment must be balanced against rapid judgments. In the study of the jnd there never is the stress of time present, since the procedures all emphasize that an individual should be as accurate as possible.

Why then should this type of judgment be studied within the context of this book? One valuable piece of information that the study of the jnd gives us is an indication of the "keenness" of a sensory system. That is, the jnd gives us a baseline measure of a sense's capacity to discriminate information, and therefore might prove to be useful when that sense is studied in detail to determine whether it really is capable of supplying information to a performer about his motor performance. For instance, it has always been felt by many people who study perceptual-motor skills that kinesthesis is an important sensory system for supplying information for the performance of these skills. If one is to find out whether this is really so, perhaps the most logical place to start is with an investigation of this system's ability to make judgments of a simple nature. Once this capacity is determined, it can then be compared to other sensory systems, which are known to be important (for example, vision), in terms of its basic "keenness." If it can be shown that kinesthesis is just as sensitive as vision, then there is a start toward the conclusion that information derived through kinesthesis can be discriminated in a manner comparable to that of other acute senses. In actual fact, this is exactly what will be done in a later section of this chapter, entitled "Information Comparison and Absolute Judgment of Kinesthetic Information."

Before leaving this topic of Information Comparison, however, some space will be given to discussing how different sensory systems can be compared in their ability to judge differences in information intensities. As established previously, the jnd is a measure of how keen a sense is, but there are two problems with the use of this measure. First, a jnd is expressed in measurement units specific to the type of information from which it was derived. Thus, we cannot compare a jnd derived from visual brightness, which is expressed in photons, to a jnd derived from lifted weights (sometimes used to measure kinesthetic sensitivity), which is measured in grams. Second, another problem might be that the jnd established through the use of one standard might be different from the jnd measured from a more intense standard. An example of this would be a jnd for a standard weight of 300 gm compared to one for a standard of 10 lb. Obviously, the jnd for the former standard will be much smaller than that of the latter.

Both of the above problems are resolved when one considers Weber's law. Weber, a German physiologist, found that for most sensory systems the amount of information change that can be detected as jnd is approximately proportional to the intensity of the standard. Thus, his law is expressed as the ratio:

$$K = \frac{\Delta I}{I}$$

where K is a constant, ΔI is the jnd, and I is the intensity of the standard. If we apply Weber's law to our example of lifting weights, we can see that to be jnd the standard weights (that is, 300 gm and 10 lb) would have to be increased by a constant fraction. If this constant were, let us say 0.2, then the 300-gm standard would have to be increased by 60 gm and the 10-lb standard would have to be increased by 2 lb in order for an individual to judge the resulting comparison weights (that is, 360 gm and 12 lb) as jnd from their respective standards. As Woodworth and Schlosberg (1954) demonstrate, the Weber constant does accurately describe most sensory systems, in terms of the jnd, especially for the middle ranges of intensity. However, the Weber constant varies markedly between different sensory systems and represents the discriminating powers of the various senses. The smaller the Weber constant the keener the sense. In addition, since the Weber constant is dimensionless (the specific units of measurement were eliminated by the division of ΔI by I), constants obtained from different senses are directly comparable. Figure 8 presents Weber constants and, as can be seen, the keenest sense is that of discriminating pitch, with a constant of 0.003. The lifting of weights, which is sometimes used as a measure of kinesthetic sensitivity, has a constant of 0.019 and falls between the Weber ratios for visual brightness and loudness, which indicates a fair degree of sensitivity.

Pitch, at 2000 Hz	0.003
Sup pressure, at 400 gm	0.013
Visual brightness, at 1000 photons	0.016
Lifted weights, at 300 gm	0.019
Loudness, at 1000 Hz, 100 dB	0.088
Smell, rubber, at 200 olfactics	0.101
Cutaneous pressure, spot, at 5 gm/mm^2	0.136
Taste, saline, at 3 moles per liter	0.200

FIGURE 8 Minimal Weber fractions (from Woodworth and Schlosberg, 1954, p. 223).

Absolute Judgment (Recognition)

Absolute judgments are similar to comparative judgments in that both involve comparing a standard stimulus with a test or comparison stimulus. However, absolute judgment is different in that the standard is not physically present but is in the memory of the individual making the judgment. In essence, information must be classified or recognized based on a comparison between it and a representation of that information in memory. A simple example of an absolute judgment task would be to judge the loudness of tones by assigning numbers to them as they were individually presented. The listener would have previously learned which number went with which tone by the number and tone being presented together. For example, if there were five different tones, with the lowest being one and the highest five, each tone would be presented with its corresponding number until the listener was sure he knew what tone went with what number. The tones would then be individually and randomly presented and the listener would have to identify it by number. Although this type of judgment seems to be relatively easy, this experiment using five tones was conducted by Pollack (1952) and there were a considerable number of errors committed by the subject.

Before describing the results of other studies concerned with absolute judgment, more information is needed on the methodology used in them. The typical experiment will start with only two or three stimuli; the subjects will learn a correct response to them (like a number); and then just the stimuli will be randomly and individually presented, and the subject must attempt to identify the stimuli by assigning the correct number to them. After this is done, a larger number of stimuli are used, perhaps five, and the learning and testing procedure repeated. The number of stimuli, over the course of the total experiment, are slowly increased in increments of about two or three to a number of around twenty.

The purpose of the absolute judgment experiment is to determine the capacity of the recognition process within the perceptual mechanism. For this purpose, the perceptual mechanism is again likened to an information channel that has an information input and an output. For absolute judgment the information input is the number of stimuli used and the output is the subject's response in attempting to identify the stimuli. Remembering that information is equivalent to uncertainty, one can see that the absolute judgment experiment varies uncertainty or information by starting with only a few stimuli (low information input) and slowly increasing the number to a substantial amount (high information input). If the channel has an unlimited capacity to process information, one would expect that there would be a one-to-one correspondence between the information input and the output. That is to say, the subject would make no errors. This relationship is described in Figure 9, where there is a perfect relationship between input and output information. However, if the channel has a limited capacity, one would expect that a point would be reached whereby increasing the amount of input information would cause only errors and the number of correct responses would level off at the capacity of the channel. This relationship is depicted in Figure 9, where in up to about 6 stimuli there are no mistakes, but beyond this point increasing the number of input stimuli only causes errors to be made, with the number of correct responses remaining roughly the same. The highest number of correct responses would be the channel capacity for that particular judgment task.

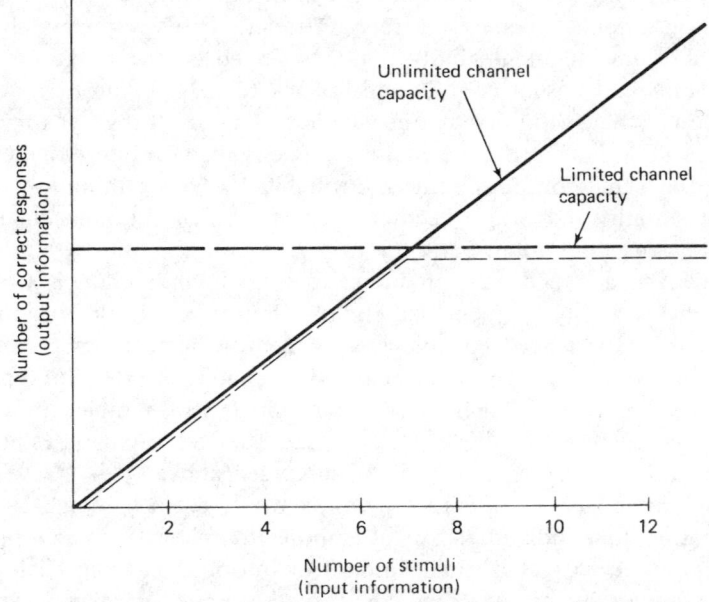

FIGURE 9 An illustration of the limited channel capacity for absolute judgments.

What is the channel capacity of individuals making absolute judgments? Surprisingly, it is very limited. Miller (1956), in a paper entitled "The Magical Number Seven, Plus or Minus Two: Some Limits on Our Capacity for Processing Information," summarized a very large amount of evidence indicating that the judgment of stimuli along a single sensory continuum was quite restricted. The types of stimuli investigated were tones, saltiness, visual positions, and visual judgments about the curvature, length, and direction of lines. Miller found that from all these experiments the average number of alternative stimuli that would be distinguished correctly was 6.5, with the range of 4 to 10 stimuli representing plus or minus one standard deviation from the mean. The total range of the number of correct stimuli, which represents the channel capacity, was from 3 to 15 stimuli. Miller concludes by stating that, considering the wide variety of stimuli studied, these figures represent a very narrow range, which demonstrates the limitation of the ability to make absolute judgments.

These limitations appear even more remarkable if one compared absolute judgment ability to information comparison ability, as discussed in the preceding section of this chapter. The small Weber constants presented for various stimuli indicate that man can virtually discriminate hundreds of different stimuli along one sensory continuum as long as both standard and comparison stimuli are simultaneously present. However, once the standard is required to be kept in memory, the ability to identify comparison stimuli becomes severely restricted. It also appears that this limited absolute judgment ability is little affected by the range of stimuli used, as Fitts and Posner (1967) and Pollack (1952) point out. The latter author found that it did not matter whether he used a range of tones over 250 Hz or 8000 Hz, in that the channel capacity for absolute judgment was roughly the same for both ranges. Probably the only limitation on the range of stimuli used would be the requirement that the adjacent stimuli along a sensory continuum be at least one jnd apart.

Since the above discussion indicates that an individual is quite restricted in his ability to recognize stimuli along a single dimension, how is it that the experienced ball player can identify many types of different information about thrown or hit balls that enables him to hit or catch successfully. Individuals, then, when confronted with complex perceptual information seem not to be limited by the channel capacity established for the simple one-dimensional stimuli discussed above.

The answer to this apparent paradox would seem to come from the consideration that individuals, in attempting to recognize a complex information input, extract a small amount of information from each of the various stimulus dimensions that comprise the input. An experiment that demonstrates this principle was completed by Pollack (1952). In this experiment he asks subjects to judge a tone both by its loudness and pitch. He found that the channel capacity for this task was a little over 8 different stimuli, which exceeded both the capacity for loudness alone (about 5 stimuli) and pitch alone (about 5.5 stimuli). Thus it appeared that his subjects somehow combined the two dimensions of pitch and loudness to increase the channel capacity for absolute judgment. It is important to note, however, that the resulting capacity was somewhat less than what would have been expected if subjects merely added together the information from pitch and loudness to make their judgments. If this were the case they should have been able to make about 10 or 11 correct judgments. That this did not occur indicates that by combining different dimensions to make complex absolute judgments, the overall channel capacity is increased, but at the expense of a decreased accuracy for any single sensory dimension that comprises the multidimensional stimulus. There have been several other studies, summarized by Miller (1956) and Fitts and Posner (1967), that demonstrate the same trend as indicated above, thus serving to validate the generality of this finding.

What this means, as expressed by Grossman (1964), is that recognition of very complex stimuli proceeds by the observer extracting a little information from each of the many stimulus dimensions that comprise the stimulus. In this way enough information is acquired that can allow accurate recognition. Thus for the recognition of one face among many, information is derived from nose length, eye color, hair color and style, ear size, and so on, until enough information is acquired that allows recognition to be made. Similarly, one can argue that in complex sport situations an individual recognizes certain events by attending to a complex array of cues and by acquiring a little information from each cue and thereby he is able to add these separate sources of information together to form a basis for recognition. One can appreciate the perceptual ability of a highly skilled tennis player who "reads" many cues from his opponent in order to recognize or identify the speed and placement of a returned ball.

Detection, Comparison, and Absolute Judgment of Kinesthetic Information

The three preceding sections of this chapter have dealt with relatively simple processes that can limit information processing within the perceptual mechanism. Information detection, comparison, and absolute judgment abilities were all discussed in terms of how they limit the capacity to transmit information through the perceptual mechanism. The former two abilities, as was discussed, can be thought of as measuring the keenness of a sensory system in terms of its ability to "pick up" information. Absolute judgment, however, represents a different kind of ability in that it involves comparing sensory information to memory.

The purpose of this section will be to study the above three processes in terms of how they limit an individual's ability to process kinesthetic information. Kinesthetic information, in terms of the model presented in Figure 2, can be thought of as information derived from the movement of our muscles and joints that is fed back to the perceptual mechanism and must be sensed, compared, and identified in a manner similar to information derived from the environment. To this extent, kinesthesis can be more broadly thought of as one aspect of knowledge of performance, which represents information that must be processed in an identical manner to all other input information. Since the control and learning of motor performance depends on feedback, and kinesthesis is one very important source of feedback about performance, it would seem important to know something about the basic sensory capacities of this system. To this end, this section is devoted to understanding the capacities of a performer for detecting, comparing, and recognizing kinesthetic information.

Definition of Kinesthesis and Its Sensory Receptors

Howard and Templeton (1966) have suggested that kinesthesis includes the discrimination of movement and amplitude of movement of body parts, both passively and actively produced. Though eliminating visual, auditory, and verbal information from kinesthesis, they believe that afferents from muscles, tendons, and ligaments—as well as touch, stretch, and pressure receptors—subsume this sense. Keele (1968) believes that the pattern or sequence of motor commands, sometimes called efference, also acts as a source of kinesthetic information. Other reviews, while sometimes slightly changing this definition of kinesthesis (some eliminate touch and pressure receptors from the definition), all present a similar viewpoint, and the serious reader is encouraged to read them to acquire a detailed description of this sense (Keele, 1968; Smith, 1969; Marteniuk and Hayes, 1975).

To broaden the understanding of the kinesthetic system some knowledge about the receptors that are sensitive to movement is necessary. A variety of sensory nerve endings are activated by the angular displacement of a body part. The Ruffini organs, contained in the ligamentous capsules surrounding joints, signal position or location information (Eldred, 1967) and are differentially excited at different joint angles. Velocity of movement, on the other hand, is signaled by receptors called muscle spindles. Muscle spindles, diagrammed in Figure 10, are found throughout the mass of the muscle, but tend to be concentrated in the central portion. The fact that there are more spindles in an individual's manipulative muscles than in his postural muscles indicates the important role of muscle spindles in precise, manipulative movements. The stimulus for these receptors is muscle stretch, and they have two basic components to their response. One component, arising from the primary nerve endings (annulospiral endings), yields a dynamic response in that they signal velocity of stretch as well as amount of stretch. The second component, consisting of activity arising from the secondary endings (flower sprays), responds only to amount of stretch. However, in addition to these two components, recent research (Goodwin, McCloskey, and Matthews, 1972) has shown that muscle spindles may also be capable of providing information about limb position. This view of muscle spindles having conscious representation contrasts with earlier conclusions of Merton (1964) and various other researchers (Brindley and Merton, 1960; Mountcastle and Powell, 1954).

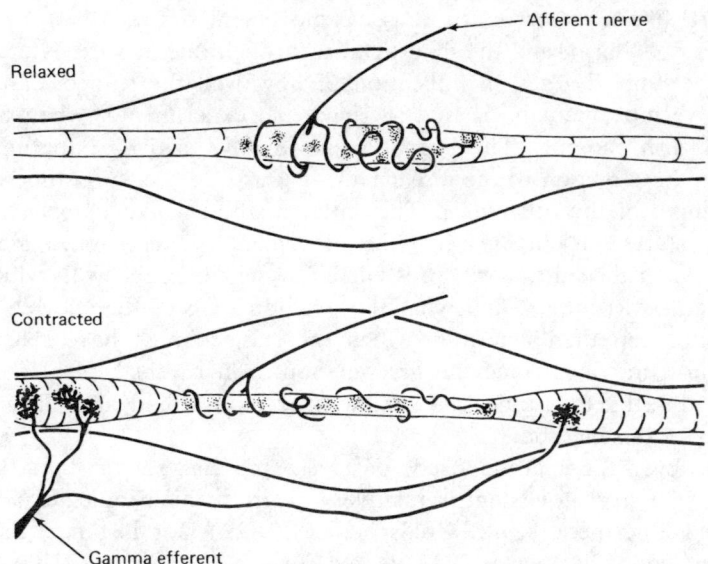

FIGURE 10 The muscle spindle. From E. Eldred, The dual sensory role of muscle spindles, chapter in *The Child with Central Nervous System Deficit*. Washington, D.C.: U.S. Dept. of Health, Education and Welfare, Children's Bureau Publication No. 432, 1965.

One other important source of kinesthetic information is derived from the acceleration of a limb. However, this information cannot be separated from that of force, since force is equal to the product of mass and acceleration. As a consequence, any force applied to a limb will result in a predictable change in its acceleration or change in velocity. Thus, the acceleration of a limb could conceivably be signaled by receptors that monitor the rate of change of velocity or those monitoring force. Both types of signals have been shown to exist in that Eldred (1967) has indicated that Ruffini organs yield a small response to acceleration, and Houk and Henneman (1967) have documented the fact that Golgi tendon organs monitor tension within a muscle.

Detection of Passive Movement

It seems from the above that the human body is well equipped to discriminate movements of its body parts. Just how accurate are these judgments? To determine this, we leave the neurological description of kinesthesis and turn to behavioral research investigating the detection ability of kinesthesis. The main method used to study detection of movement necessarily involves the detection of passive movement of a limb or limb part, like a finger or toe. Passive movement occurs when a subject relaxes, say his arm, and the investigator, through one of various methods, moves the limb. To get an indication of how well the subject can sense the passive movement he is told to signal the experimenter when he first feels his arm moving. This signal could involve actively stopping and reversing the direction of the movement or pressing a reaction time button with a finger of the other arm. This latter method would involve a clock that was started at the onset of the movement of the passive arm and stopped when the button was pressed. Knowing the speed with which the passive arm was moved and what the reaction time of the subject is, the investigator can then determine when the subject must have sensed his passive arm moving. Since the first method, arm reversal, also implies a reaction time by the subject, a similar procedure would also have to be followed for this method.

Whatever the method used, past research has shown that the detection of passive movement is relatively precise, which indicates a highly developed kinesthetic sense. Goldscheider (1889), for instance, reported threshold values as low as 0.22 degree for the shoulder and hip joints. Although the thresholds for various different joints varied somewhat, they all indicated keen sensitivity. In similar investigations, Pillsbury (1901) and Winter (1912) reported threshold values that were as low as 0.20 degree, with none exceeding 0.85 degree. Results from more recent investigations support these earlier studies (Cleghorn and Darcus, 1952; Davies, 1966).

Active Movement

One drawback to studying passive movement is that in perceptual-motor skills most movement is actively produced. That is, a performer sees a need for a movement and proceeds to organize and initiate it. One might ask whether the kinesthetic feedback received from this type of movement is the same as that received from passive movement. Most certainly it is not. For a start, active movement in perceptual-motor skills usually involves body and limb speeds much greater than those used in studying passive movement. Along with these greater speeds, there is greater stress put on the joints and greater muscle tension developed in the muscles. In addition, active movement also has the advantage of being initiated voluntarily so that the performer has some idea in advance as to what type of feedback to expect. This expectation could actually facilitate the reception of feedback, making it more precise than if it were from passive movement.

In studying active movement, one cannot study detection ability since the movement is self-initiated. Therefore, to determine the sensitivity of kinesthesis derived from active movement the method of information comparison has to be used. The method of information comparison was used by Marteniuk, Shields, and Campbell (1972) in an attempt to determine the sensitivity of the kinesthetic system so that it could be compared to that of other sensory systems. Using the Method of Average Error (Woodworth and Schlosberg, 1954) the task of the subject was actively to move a lever, pivoted on near frictionless ball bearings, until the lever hit a block. This defined the standard movement. The subject then returned the lever to the starting position and immediately attempted to reproduce the standard movement, but this time without the aid of the block. The experimenter then recorded the error of the reproduction, which was the end point of the reproduction movement minus the end point of the standard movement. The presentation of a standard and its reproduction was called a trial, and each of 10 subjects was given 100 trials for each of three different standard movements. These standard movements represented movement lengths of 45 degrees, 90 degrees, and 125 degrees.

The results of this investigation produced just noticeable differences of 1.95 degrees, 2.20 degrees, and 2.13 degrees for each of the three standards, respectively, which were significantly different from each other. These figures were not significantly different from each other and represented Weber ratios of .043, .024, and .017, respectively. Two aspects of these results prove to be interesting in attempts to define the sensory characteristics of kinesthesis. First, from the previous discussion of the Weber ratios (in the section on information comparison), it was shown that for most sensory systems this ratio is a constant. In other words, the just noticeable difference for a weak standard would be much smaller than the corresponding figure for a more intense standard. This characteristic of other sensory systems obviously does not hold for kinesthesis. Rather, it appears from the above results that the just noticeable difference is a constant. These results are explainable if one considers the type of receptors that provide information concerned with the judgments in the lever positioning task that was used by Marteniuk, Shields, and Campbell. If it can be assumed that the receptors within the joints play a prominent role in providing relevant information about limb position it would be reasonable to suppose that different limb positions were signaled by different populations of receptors. In other words it seems that the type of kinesthetic receptor involved in discrimination of movement is a qualitative receptor mechanism. Thus one would expect that discrimination of movement would be the same for one population of receptors as for another. The kinesthetic sensory system is almost unique in this way, although those receptors involved in the discrimination of pitch function in a similar manner. Most other sensory systems are characterized by quantitative receptor mechanisms in which different intensities of a stimulus are signaled by the number of receptors fired. Thus receptors involved in signaling weak stimuli are also involved in signaling more intense stimuli, with the only difference being that for the latter stimuli there are more receptors. It is senses that are served by these types of receptor systems that follow Weber's law. This is logical in that for weak stimuli only a few receptors are activated, and for a second stimulus to be just noticeably different there need be only a relatively few more receptors activated. However, if there is an intense stimulus that fires thousands of receptors, then another stimulus will have to be quite a bit more intense in order for enough additional receptors to be fired that a difference in receptor activity can be discriminated.

Even though it appears that position sense may not follow Weber's law, the second interesting finding of the Marteniuk, Shields, and Campbell study was that feedback from active movement provides relatively precise information for arm positioning. The three Weber ratios reported all fall between the Weber ratios for visual brightness (0.016) and loudness (0.088) as reported in Woodworth and Schlosberg (1954), indicating that kinesthesis is at least as sensitive as the two so-called dominant senses.

The evidence presented so far, then, indicates that detection and comparison of kinesthetic information can be carried out at a high level of preciseness. Evidently, the kinesthetic system is just as capable of supplying sensory information to the perceptual mechanism as are the senses of vision and audition. However, this does not imply that this kinesthetic information can be used for more complex perceptual judgments. One type of judgment that is more complex than detection and comparison abilities is absolute judgment, and it will be fruitful to consider whether kinesthesis can be used on a par with other sensory systems in this type of information processing task.

Absolute Judgment

Absolute judgment is a more complex perceptual task than information detection or comparison because its success depends on memory. As discussed previously, there are definite limitations on the ability to compare a stimulus to memory for such tasks as identifying auditory tones and identifying visual positions. Certainly, however, absolute judgment underlies a large part of information processing of visual and auditory information in the perceptual mechanism.

It can be argued as well that absolute judgment of kinesthetic information may play a large part in the performance and learning of perceptual-motor skills. To understand where absolute judgment may be important, it is necessary to first understand the closed-loop theory of motor learning. Adams (1971) has recently set forth a theory of motor learning based upon closed-loop concepts. At the base of all closed-loop mechanisms is a standard that serves as a reference to be compared to current feedback from some operation. A good example of motor performance involving closed-loop control is driving a car. Here the standard might simply be to keep the car on the right-hand side of the road. Through visual feedback the driver determines whether or not he is achieving this standard and, if he is not (he could be driving on the centerline), he must perform some operation (a motor act) to correct the perceived discrepancy. Once he has carried out his correction, he must once again sample his visual feedback to determine whether the standard was achieved. If it was achieved, he would still periodically have to compare visual feedback to the standard to note any discrepancies due to a winding road, wandering of the car, or some unplanned movement of the steering wheel. This closed-loop process is diagrammed in Figure 11.

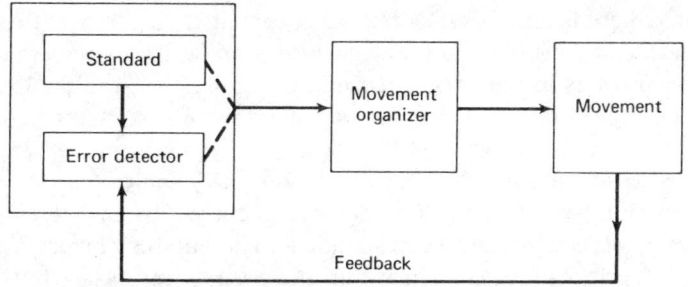

FIGURE 11   A closed-loop control system.

Adams (1971) believes that a type of closed-loop mechanism underlies motor performance and learning. At the base of his theory are two habit states. One of these he calls the memory trace, which fires the motor response when its stimulus occurs. The other is called the perceptual trace, and it is the image of environmental and response-produced stimuli, a large part of which is kinesthetic in origin, which acts as an individual's reference level when determining the appropriatenes of a response. In essence, the correctness of the response is determined by the comparison of the feedback from that response to the perceptual trace.

The important point of the above description of the closed-loop theory of motor learning is that it predicts that for successful motor performance to occur there must be a comparison between a memory of movement (the perceptual trace) and current kinesthetic feedback, which is an absolute judgment. It becomes important then to determine whether a performer is actually capable of making absolute judgments involving kinesthetic information. If the theory is correct, it should eventually be shown that the channel capacity for recognition of kinesthetic information should be on a par with those of other sensory systems.

To date, only two studies have been completed in this area of study. Marteniuk (1971) investigated the ability of subjects to recognize kinesthetic feedback resulting from active movements of varying lengths. In essence, he conducted five experiments in which the subjects in each experiment learned the relationship between different movement lengths and the number assigned to them. For instance, in the first experiment four different movement lengths were used. Subjects moved a level until it hit a block, which designated the end of the movement, and the subject was then told that this was either movement length 1, 2, 3, or 4, with movement 1 being the shortest and movement 4 being the longest. Subjects were given as much practice as they wanted in this phase of the experiment. In the test phase of the experiment the subject then had to move the lever until it was stopped by the block and then he had to tell the experimenter what movement length it was—that is, movement 1, 2, 3, or 4. Presumably, the subject at this point had well-formed standards or perceptual traces of the movements in memory and could recognize the kinesthetic feedback from each movement. In the other four experiments, subjects had to learn and then attempt to recognize 6, 8, 10, and 16 different movements.

The results of the study showed that the channel capacity, or the maximum number of correct responses, occurred when fifteen different movements were used and corresponded to about six correct judgments. There was perfect accuracy when four movements were used, but accuracy was less than perfect for all other numbers of movements. In terms of the main purpose of the study, it was concluded that the kinesthetic sense can provide precise information for the recognition of movement. The capacity of this system would seem to be on a par with the ability of other senses to provide information on an absolute basis in that six correct judgments fall well within Miller's (1956) "Magical number seven plus or minus two" capacity noted for a wide variety of absolute judgment tasks.

Another study concerned with absolute judgment of kinesthetic information is one by Russell and Marteniuk (1974). Instead of investigating feedback from movement extent, they concentrated on another important source of information for movement, namely force cues. Whenever an individual voluntarily moves his body or a limb, there is of necessity some tension developed in the muscles and tendons and, as discussed previously, information about tension or force is signaled by the Golgi tendon organs. The question is, however, whether a performer can recognize different levels of tension accurately. If he can, it would indicate that this type of information might be usable in the control and learning of movements.

Russell and Marteniuk in essence followed the same procedures as established by Marteniuk (1971) in that they looked at accuracy of recognition of force in experiments that gradually increased the total number of different force levels. They found that the channel capacity for force was a little lower than that for movement extent in that the maximum number of correct responses was about 3½ levels of force. This number still represents a level of judgment that is at least equal to several other sensory systems.

The next step in the investigation of absolute judgment of kinesthetic information is to examine multidimensional kinesthetic cues. This would undoubtedly be difficult from a procedural point of view but it would prove fruitful to determine whether performers are capable of more accurate judgments about movement when they have various types of kinesthetic cues simultaneously present. For a starter, force and movement extent cues could be combined and the channel capacity for recognition could be determined. If kinesthesis is like other sensory systems, the channel capacity should be increased over what it was for force and movement extent separately, but not as much as would be expected by just adding together the maximum number of correct judgments from each of these cues.

Selective Attention

The fact that a performer can detect, compare, and recognize information does not necessarily imply that he will be able to attend to the information relevant to the successful performance of a skill. It may be, for instance, that a tennis player attends to the wrong information when attempting to track a ball just hit by his opponent. Although he has initially processed these signals, they are not appropriate to the true flight characteristics of the ball, and as a result he will be unable to play the ball successfully. Gentile (1972) labels the information of the display that dictates how a successful motor response must be organized and executed as regulatory information, and all other information as nonregulatory or irrelevant. The question of what psychological factors enable a performer to distinguish between regulatory and nonregulatory information is the concern of this section on selective attention.

In Chapter 3 of this book three aspects of the broad term "attention" were defined. It will be seen that the treatment of selective attention embodies the concept of the other two aspects of attention, namely alertness and the limited information processing channel. Without an optimal level of arousal, efficient information processing could not take place in terms of selecting certain types of information over other types. At the same time, it will be seen that information selection can take part of or, at times, all of the limited information processing capacity of an individual's central nervous system. Therefore, it might be said that perception is limited by attention in three ways: alertness, information processing capacity, and information selection. We now turn to a discussion of how this latter process limits information processing within the perceptual mechanism.

In any skill situation the relevant information in the environment must be attended to so that further processing of the information can proceed. How does the individual selectively attend to the relevant information at the exclusion of irrelevant information? This aspect of behavior is called *selective attention*, and it is the process whereby attention is focused on certain aspects of the environment, with perception the end result. Selective attention is necessary because of the limited information processing capacity of the central nervous system, which is incapable of attending to or processing all aspects of the environment, and therefore only certain aspects of this information must be selected. A point worth mentioning right now is that a person performing an open perceptual-motor skill not only must be concerned with selecting information from the environment but also must attend to the feedback (both knowledge of performance and knowledge of results) from his performance. Thus the performer's task is a complex one in that he not only must select the correct information from the environment that tells him how to respond, but he also must be prepared to receive and select appropriate feedback from his response so that he can determine how successful it was. This direct selection of environmental and feedback information is made even more complex when one considers that most skills are continuous in nature, so the two streams of information are continually overlapping with each other. This process is diagrammed in Figure 12, which shows the perceptual mechanism receiving three distinct sources of information, which would sometimes be simultaneous, at other times overlapping, and in some cases sequential.

How well does an individual process information from more than two sources when it is received simultaneously? The whole point of this section

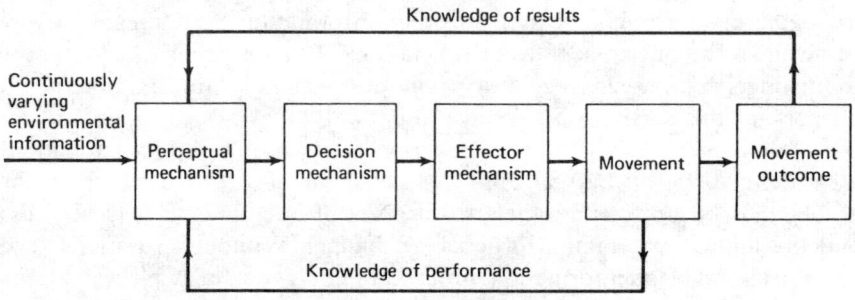

FIGURE 12   Information processing in an open skill.

on selective attention is to show that the individual with little or no experience in specific situations will be tremendously handicapped in processing the relevant information from this situation. On the other hand, the individual who has had a lot of experience with the specific information somehow overcomes this handicap and it appears that he can process all the pertinent information received by his sensory systems. By the end of this section it should be apparent why this is the case.

To understand how well an individual can attend to two sources of simultaneously presented information we can turn to the work of Cherry (1953). He likens the study of selective attention to the phenomenon that occurs at a cocktail party. He reasons that a cocktail party is a good place to study selective attention because there are usually many different simultaneous messages that a listener is presented with. One example of a situation at a cocktail party that illustrates one aspect of selective attention is when a listener is extremely interested in the conversation of one individual. Even if the talker is not speaking very loudly and even if there is considerable noise from other people talking, the listener is able to shut out all the irrelevant noise and "zero in" or attend to the conversation of interest. It is as if he is capable of blocking or filtering out all irrelevant information. However, while fully attending to this conversation, if from somewhere else in the room the listener's name is mentioned, this "message" somehow gets through the filters that had previously blocked out all other information except that from the speaker of interest. Thus even though the listener was paying no attention to the source of information from which his name occurred, somehow it was able to gain access to the limited information processing channel and be processed.

Since a cocktail party is not a good place to carry out well-controlled experiments, Cherry (1953) devised an experimental task that allowed him to study the perception of information when two messages were presented simultaneously to an individual. His task was to present to a subject, through earphones, two simultaneous messages, one to his right ear and one to his left. The subject was then instructed to pay attention to the message of one ear and repeat back what he heard. After this, the subject was asked what he had heard on the unattended ear.

The results of this latter question were surprising in light of what had been presented. Cherry had designed the "unattended" message so that the central or major aspect of it involved: (1) normal English speech spoken by a male; (2) a change from a message spoken in English to one spoken in German; (3) a change from a male voice to a female voice; (4) a change from normal speech to reversed speech; and (5) a change from speech to a 400-Hz pure tone. In answer to what the subjects had heard on the unattended ear, the responses for each of the above situations, respectively were: (1) subjects knew that there was a message being presented but they were unable to identify any words or phrases from it; (2) the change from English to German was not noticed; (3) the change from a male voice to a female voice was noticed; (4) the reversed speech was noticed by some subjects in that they only thought something was different about the message, while for most subjects the reversed speech went unnoticed; and (5) the pure tone was almost always observed.

The results of this study indicate that individuals are severely limited in their ability to attend to simultaneously presented information to their central nervous systems. As long as attention is on one source of information, recall is good; but if a message is not attended to, only certain aspects of the message, such as one's name or a change from a male to female voice, tend to be recognized.

If individuals are severely restricted in attending to simultaneously presented information, what are the implications for perceptual-motor performance? The limitation imposed by selective attention seems to account for the performance of very inexperienced performers like a novice basketball player in his first game. The many stimuli competing for his attention include: the feedback he is receiving from his own actions, which in all likelihood represents a great deal of uncertainty; the information necessary to coordinate his actions with those of his teammates; the information he must process regarding the action of his opponents; and the necessity, on occasion, to plan and execute some movement in an offensive or defensive play. Cherry's (1953) work on selective attention tells us that a novice will be unable to attend simultaneously to all sources of information and may indeed be able to attend to only one source of information. It is no wonder that the novice player makes so many mistakes, and the mistakes he is making, in the context of this discussion, are the result of perceptual limitations imposed by limitations in selective attention.

However, why does this limitation on the perceptual ability of a novice player not appear to hold for the very experienced one? It certainly seems that the skilled basketball player attends to all relevant information, so that from a perceptual viewpoint he is able to process all relevant information from the various sources mentioned previously in the description of the information sources faced by a novice player. Before an answer to this question can be given, a review of the major selective attention theories is necessary.

A simplified version of a model of selective attention presented by Broadbent (1958) is illustrated in Figure 13. Although he attempted to specify the underlying processes of attention only in regard to the recognition of speech, the principle of his model can be adapted to meet the needs for analyzing perceptual-motor performance. Central to his model was the idea that somewhere in the central nervous system there exists a limited capacity channel (that is, a single communication channel). Since the

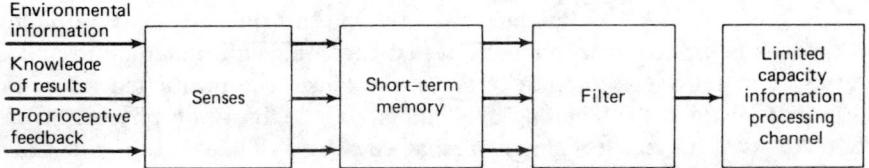

FIGURE 13 A simplified version of Broadbent's (1958) selective attention model.

input to the central nervous system was seen as multichanneled, where a channel can be thought of as an input from a sensory receptor, it was therefore necessary to postulate the presence of filters (selective attention), which performed a selective function on the input and only allowed the most pertinent information access to the limited capacity channel. This operation was necessary in order to avoid "jamming" the single channel. These filters were seen as selecting information by physical features such as intensity, pitch, and spatial location of sounds. Selection of information was also guided by certain properties of the events, such as their probability of occurrence and the time that the information last entered the limited capacity channel. In order that nonselected information could still be processed by the limited capacity channel, Broadbent postulated a short-term store, located prior to the filter, for the input information that was not initially selected. Thus once the limited capacity channel had processed the initial or high-priority information, it could process additional information contained in the short-term memory store. This memory was seen as also being limited by time, with a maximum time for storage of the order of seconds. Nevertheless, it had the potential of acting as a buffer between the high level of input information and the rather limited processing capacity. Finally Broadbent indicated that switching of the filter among different input channels took a finite period of time and thus limited the selection of information.

Although Broadbent's model stimulated a great amount of research that contributed toward an understanding of attention, it was eventually found to be lacking. The major shortcoming was the model's inability to explain how information on unattended channels sometimes reached the limited capacity channel. Subjectively, this is seen in a situation where an individual is actively attending to one source of information, perhaps concentrating on something a friend is saying, and then hears his name mentioned by someone else who is not only some distance removed but is only talking in a normal voice. According to Broadbent, this should not happen, since all information is selected by the physical characteristics of the message. In essence, the model failed because it failed to account for selection of information through meaningfulness of the information in unattended channels.

Treisman (1964) attempted to overcome this difficulty by postulating a type of filter that hierarchically tested incoming information through a series of increasingly complex tests. At the outset she postulated an initial test that distinguished among the inputs on the basis of physical cues. Later tests distinguished among verbal cues by syllabic patterns, specific sounds, individual words, and last, through grammatical structure and meaning. Expectations of certain words or phrases enhanced the passage of those signals by biasing the tests in favor of those signals. Finally, a word that was initially filtered or attenuated might still gain access to the limited capacity channel if later tests indicated that the words fitted into the context or meaning of material just analyzed. In addition, Treisman believed that some words or groups of words (like a person's name, danger signals, or words that were highly contextually probable) had permanently lowered thresholds for activation so that when they occurred in the environment they were immediately attended to. Thus, Treisman offers some degree of flexibility in her model by postulating lowered thresholds for important words and by increasing the complexity of the filter in terms of the number of tests that words or sentences are submitted to. However, according to Norman (1969) this is the downfall of the model. He reasons that Treisman's model is too complex, since it in essence predicts that all input information is analyzed to a great degree and in this way the model loses its power of selectivity. That is, the model failed to show how man efficiently reduces the vast amount of input information to a few relevant alternatives for processing by the limited capacity channel.

To overcome the difficulties encountered by the Broadbent and Treisman models, Norman (1969) has presented a model (Figure 14) that differs in a number of ways from the previous two.

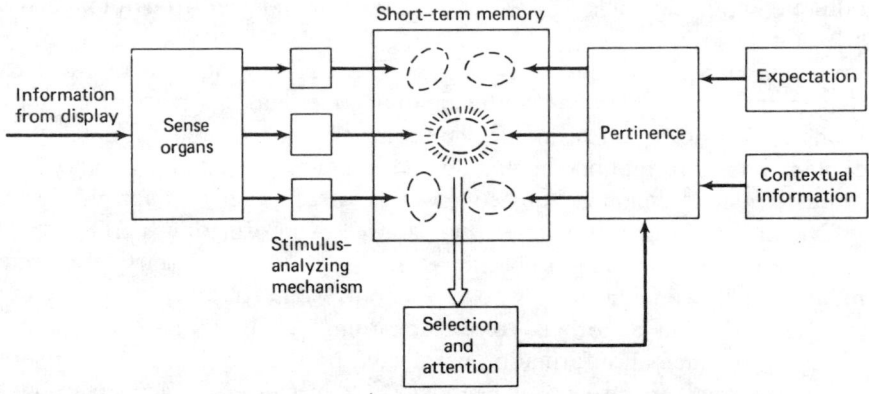

FIGURE 14 Norman's (1969) selective attention model. From Norman, 1969.

According to Norman, the process of selectively attending to a stimulus, which results in recognition of that information, entails a number of information processing stages. Starting at the sensory end, the sensory receptors within the sense organs code the information from the display. This information is then passed to a set of physiological stimulus-analyzing mechanisms that extract important parameters for further analysis. These parameters then excite their stored representation in memory and the result is that these representations are stored temporarily in short-term memory. It is important to note that Norman postulates that this total process demands none of the performer's attention (or space, as defined in Chapter 3), and the implication is that the excitation of memory by stimuli entering through the sense organs is done automatically. Because it requires no attention, the performer, for this particular process, can also be described as a "parallel" processor in that information from all sense organs can be processed in parallel or simultaneously. The only limitation to this process would be one of time in that it would take some finite time period (of the order of milliseconds) for information from the display to be coded, analyzed, and then excite its representation in memory.

While the analysis of sensory information is going on, an equally important analysis is proceeding as indicated by the right-hand side of Figure 14. According to Norman, another set of memorial representations is excited (but this time by the performer's expectations), and information is derived from contextual cues that combine to give the performer a set of pertinent events that he believes to be most appropriate for the particular situation with which he is confronted. That is, through past experience, the performer is able to "ready" or excite in memory a class of events that he believes to be most pertinent to the analysis of information from the display. Expectations of events can be seen as being derived from past experience in which the performer can assign probabilities to events in terms of their likelihood of actually occurring in a particular situation. Contextual cues, likewise, also depend on past experience, but here a performer makes use of the context in which an event occurs to establish pertinence for a particular class of events. An example of how a performer uses contextual cues in a perceptual motor skill would be a batter attempting to recognize the type of pitch being delivered by a pitcher. It may be that the batter, by watching the way the pitcher winds up and releases the ball (that is, the context of the pitch) will be able to decide which kind of pitch is most likely. This information plus that gained from the batter's expectations before the pitcher wound up (for example, the count is 3 and 2 and the pitcher likes to throw a fast ball in this situation) go together to excite in memory those events deemed most important to the ongoing analysis.

According to Norman, and as illustrated in Figure 14, the item that is selectively attended to is that item most highly excited by the combination of sensory and pertinence inputs. It stands to reason then that if an event occurs in the display and was also highly pertinent, it has a high probability of being selectively attended to. Selective attention here is the end result of the recognition process, with the recognized event or item being used not only for deciding upon a course of action, but also to update or refine the pertinence judgments.

Of importance in the above description of how selective attention occurs is that the excitation of items or events in memory do not require attention or space. It is only the selection of an item and the subsequent attention to it that place a demand on the performer's limited information processing capacity. Thus it is this aspect of the recognition process that serves as the bottleneck in processing perceptual information. If the selected item requires all of the performer's limited information processing capacity, he in essence becomes a sequential processor at this stage of performance. Thus, although a very large amount of information is taken in by the sense organs, initially processed by automatic analyzers, and thus used to activate the memory representations of the sensory events, because of the attention demand of selecting one of these representations only a very limited amount of information is actually attended to and recognized.

One can now appreciate how the selective attention process can serve to limit the performance of an individual. If a performer attends to the wrong set of items in the display, the fact that this process takes a considerable amount of his limited information processing capacity makes it highly unlikely that he will be able to recognize the appropriate information. An example of this can be seen in a novice basketball player who upon receiving a pass starts to dribble the ball. Attending to the act of dribbling occupies all his limited information processing capacity and as a result he is oblivious of his teammates and opponents. He will more than likely continue dribbling until he runs out of bounds or loses the ball to his opponents.

If selectively attending to an event requires a considerable part of the limited information processing capacity, why is it that highly skilled athletes seem capable of attending to all aspects of the environment? According to Norman's model in Figure 14, this can be explained by considering the right-hand side or pertinence part of the model. If an item has been classified as being highly pertinent and actually is present in the sensory information received from a performer, it will probably be selected and recognized. One characteristic of highly skilled individuals is that they, with considerable accuracy, can make predictions about which events are most probable. In addition, these performers can also gain considerable information from the context in which a skill is performed. Consider a skilled badminton player watching an opponent stroke a shuttlecock. By watching how he initiates and progresses through the stroke to just before contact is made with the shuttlecock an experienced performer can predict where the shuttlecock will be placed. This implies that proper execution of motor skills place considerable restraint on the possible and likely sequence of movements that can appear within a total movement pattern. Therefore, an experienced player can predict, from watching the initial movements of an opponent what the end result of the movement will be. Putting it in another way, it can be said that there is redundant information in a situation like this. Redundancy, used like this, means that an individual can predict the occurrence of an event from an earlier one so that when the predicted event occurs it is redundant information (that is, it carries no information load). In essence then, a skilled badminton player only has to sample information from the initial actions of his opponent and from this he can predict what the outcome of his opponent's action will be. Thus, when taking into consideration the information gained from both expectations and contextual cues, the information processing demand of monitoring the environment is considerably less for the experienced player. In essence he can ignore much of the input information and then, by establishing probabilities for certain events and making use of the redundancy in motor skills, he can accurately attend to the one or two items or events that are most pertinent to his successful performance.

Harry Kay (1970, p. 141) explains the influence of expectations and contextual information in selective attention when he considers the difference between the performances of children and adults. He says:

If we consider a child's performance only in terms of the known world of the adult, then often its difficulties are not apparent. But when we consider it from a child's point of view where so much is unknown and literally almost anything can happen, we begin to appreciate how much more complex is the situation for a child. It is often facing possibilities which the adult has ruled out of consideration, because on the basis of his previous experience, he can say that some events, or classes of events, are most unlikely. A child who lacks this experience has to consider more eventualities, and to that extent is having to process more information.

In the same article, Kay gives another example of how highly skilled performers are able to reduce the information load on the perceptual mechanism. He gives the example of a tennis player who has to make a rapid decision about the result of how he just hit a ball. In this situation there is usually not enough time for the performer to wait and watch the results of his stroke. Rather, highly skilled players will know where the stroked ball will go just from the "feel" of the stroke. Thus, by predicting where the ball will go through the use of proprioceptive feedback, the tennis player can considerably speed up the evaluation of the outcome of his stroke in that if he had to monitor the ball through vision a considerably slower decision process would result.

Once the tennis player learns to recognize or classify the proprioceptive feedback from various shots, a second process develops that not only again speeds up the processing of information but eliminates the necessity for monitoring or selectively attending to all the proprioceptive information received from a stroke. The process is one of developing anticipation of proprioceptive feedback from a stroke that will be executed. In essence, a highly skilled player knows in advance what stroke he is going to execute and, since he has experienced many similar strokes in the past, he can anticipate how the present stroke will feel. Thus if the tennis player executes the stroke as intended, the ensuing proprioceptive feedback will carry very little information load because it carried no uncertainty (that is, the information is redundant). The result is a considerably reduced attention demand on the limited information processing capacity of the perceptual mechanism.

The fact that the experienced player has a reduced load on his perceptual mechanism does not imply that he is not monitoring all the proprioceptive feedback from the stroke. It does imply, however, that the monitoring operation takes considerably less attention and thus leaves more of the limited information capacity for other performance demands. This means then that if the tennis player executed a stroke not as intended, the feedback would differ from the anticipated feedback and it would be detected. When this is the case the performer might then have to utilize a large portion of the limited information processing capacity to monitor the outcome of the stroke.

The above description of anticipation of feedback serves to indicate how past experience can influence selective attention, as was illustrated in Norman's (1969) model in Figure 14. From this the task faced by the novice can be appreciated. Not only does he not have any pertinence to help in processing incoming information, but the execution of his responses is erratic. This means that the feedback from these responses will be highly uncertain, which adds tremendously to his overall information input. In essence, the novice is bombarded with large amounts of information and as a result he takes considerably longer to arrive at a response. If he decides to act quickly, this would mean that he has not sufficiently processed all the relevant information and it will be just a matter of chance whether his response is correct. Thus, the novice can be characterized as a performer who either takes a long time to respond correctly or who responds quickly but incorrectly. In either case, if the skill requires decisions in short intervals of time, his performance will suffer and he will likely be unsuccessful.

Short-Term Information Memory

From the introductory discussion in Chapter 1 it was established that there were three types of memory processes concerned with the short-term retention of information. These three processes are immediate information storage, short-term information memory, and operational short-term memory. Although immediate memory storage is a very important aspect of the information processing model, it will not be discussed any further because of its rather limited application to problems in perceptual-motor skills. For those interested in reading more on the details of this information storage mechanism, the books by Fitts and Posner (1967) and Keele (1973) should be read. The present section will be concerned only with those aspects of short-term memory that are pertinent to information processing in perceptual-motor skills.

To be consistent with the organization of this book, short-term information memory will be discussed in this section mainly in terms of performance. That means that we are concerned only with a performer's ability to retain information over relatively short periods of time so that he can utilize that information to help organize, execute, and evaluate his motor performance. In a later chapter we shall be more concerned with studying what processes underlie the transfer of information from short-term memory to long-term memory.

Short-Term Memory Defined

Short-term memory can be defined simply as a memory system that rapidly loses information in the absence of sustained attention of that material. It is thought to involve about the first 60 seconds following presentation of the information, after which it is either lost or transferred to long-term memory. An example illustrating some of the processes involved in short-term memory is as follows. If a sequence of 8 digits is presented to an individual at a rate of one per second, and he is asked immediately after they are all presented to recall the digits, chances are that he will make relatively few mistakes. However, if after the 8 digits are presented to him, he is required to read one or two sentences from a book, and then repeat back the 8 digits, he will likely make quite a few mistakes. This latter situation can be compared to yet another condition where, instead of having to read sentences after the 8 digits are presented, the individual is allowed to think about the digits for a period of time corresponding to the time of reading in the former condition. In this case, when he repeats back the 8 digits his performance will probably be just as good as when he repeated the digits immediately after their presentation.

This example serves to illustrate the basic short-term memory phenomenon that we are interested in. An individual is initially presented information and then given a retention interval, after which he must recall the information. The retention interval can vary in length from immediate recall, where there would be no delay between presentation and recall, to any time up to about one minute. During the retention interval, except for immediate recall, the individual can think about or actually rehearse the information presented to him, in which case he is said to be attending to the information. Alternately, either he can be made to perform an interpolated task that is unrelated to the to-be-remembered information and thus be unable to attend to the presented information, or he can be made to perform some task that is thought to interfere directly with the presented information. In either condition, the individual cannot attend to the to-be-remembered material, and any decrement in its recall can be attributed either to lack of attention during the retention interval or to direct interference from information presented during the retention interval.

It is important to distinguish between the causes of the decrements in recall due to related and unrelated interpolated tasks. When information enters short-term memory it assumes some kind of psychological structure and, if it is to be maintained, some or all of the limited processing capacity must be devoted to attending to or rehearsing that information. If an individual is required to perform an attention-demanding interpolated task during the retention interval, this task utilizes the limited processing capacity of the individual and as a result the to-be-remembered material is interfered with in that rehearsal cannot occur. However, there may also be an additional cause of interference depending on the nature of the interpolated task. If this task, when entering short-term memory, takes the same psychological structure as the to-be-remembered information structural interference occurs and recall of the to-be-remembered information is hindered. On the other hand, if the psychological structure of the interpolated task is unrelated to that of the to-be-remembered information, the only interference caused by this task would be that due to lack of rehearsal.

Considerations of short-term memory in perceptual-motor skills and teaching. If the reader cares to reflect on the foregoing examples, he can probably see situations in either the performance or teaching of perceptual-motor skills where considerations of the characteristics of short-term memory might be important. For instance, when an individual performs a skill, he receives information about how well he performed that skill from both knowledge of results and knowledge of performance. He must then utilize that information to evaluate his performance in order that he can modify his next attempt in the hope of making it more successful. If the performer were unable to retain information from his previous attempt, whether it was due to lack of opportunity to rehearse or to structural interference caused by an interpolated activity, this evaluation and the subsequent modification of performance would not be possible.

Another example of the role short-term memory has in perceptual-motor performance can be illustrated by using a teaching situation. A teacher of motor skills usually gives a demonstration of the skill he wants his students to perform plus some verbal cues to aid the student's interpretation of how to perform it. The students then must retain this information, often for a considerable time interval while they wait for their turn, before they actually attempt to perform the skill. Consideration of how well information is retained and what affects its retention in short-term memory would thus seem to be an important aspect of teaching.

The above examples illustrate the importance of an ability to retain information over short time periods. The systematic study of short-term memory is an attempt to determine what limitations there are to this retention process. The next two sections of this chapter will attempt to review some literature that suggests what these limits are. First, the capacity of the short-term memory "store" will be discussed, where the main emphasis will be on determining how much information can be initially "stored" and recalled without a decrement in recall occurring. Second, a discussion of how long material can be stored in short-term memory will center around how fast information is lost if an individual's attention or processing capacity is diverted to other information.

Capacity of Short-Term Memory

Nonmotor information. The retention of nonmotor information (for example, verbal, visual, auditory) is of interest in that this type of information undoubtedly plays a large role in performance and learning of perceptual-motor skills. If this is not already clear to the reader, it will become more so in later chapters.

The basic capacity of short-term memory is measured through the "immediate memory span." Usually, subjects are presented random single digits, letters, or objects, one at a time, and at a rate of one per second, with the number of items in any trial ranging from only a few to as many as 10 or 15. Cardozo and Leopold (1963) presented digits to their subjects in this manner and found that only about 6 digits could be repeated back without any of their subjects ever making an error. Traditionally, immediate memory span is measured as the number of items correctly reported 50 percent of the time. When this is done, and the above procedures followed, what is usually found is an average memory span of 7 or 8 items. This appears to hold for a wide number of auditory and visual stimuli.

The problem with stating that the capacity of short-term memory is 7 or 8 items is that the term "item" has not been defined. For instance, as

Fitts and Posner (1967) point out, the memory span for letters is 7 items, whereas for simple words it is 5 items. But in the retention of words many more letters are retained than the apparent capacity of 7 when they are included as individual items in a memory span experiment. Miller (1956) resolved this apparent paradox by proposing that the limit on short-term memory can be thought of in terms of numbers of chunks of information. A chunk of information would be a meaningful familiar unit, comprised of a number of smaller items, and retained as a whole. For example your home telephone number is not retained as seven separate digits, but rather the digits are chunked together into one meaningful unit. Thus, there is a definite limitation to short-term memory and it would seem, as Miller (1956) points out, to be around 7 ± 2 chunks of information (the magical number seven again!). However, one chunk of information could conceivably contain a huge amount of information. Thus the capacity for short-term memory would seem to be a matter of organizing to-be-remembered material into familiar or meaningful chunks of information so that a maximum amount of information can be retained. Miller refers to this process of organizing information into chunks as recoding. In essence, this implies that events entering into short-term memory are grouped or organized under a name or terms so that they are not remembered individually but by the new name or terms. Thus this is obviously a very powerful way of facilitating memory.

Motor information. Just as important as the retention of visual or auditory information accompanying perceptual-motor skill is the retention of what will be called motor information. Included in this type of information would be proprioception, arising from movement, as well as information concerning what a performer intended to do. This latter information has been variously called: (1) central representations of motor plans (Keele, 1968); (2) efference (von Holst, 1954); and (3) outflow information. This type of information is supposedly concerned with organizing and initiating a response, and as the signals are sent from the brain to the muscles a copy of these efferent signals are stored in the central nervous system. Thus the performer has a memory of what he intended to do.

Studies of motor short-term memory have usually been concerned with the retention of relatively simple unidirectional movements that can vary only in extent. Thus this task differs considerably from those used in visual or auditory short-term memory experiments in that in these tasks the number of items presented to the subjects can be easily varied. Although one is tempted to say that a unidirectional movement of a given extent is probably only one item, at this point it would be unwise because it is not known how many different cues from movement a subject could be attending to as he is moving. The point is, however, that it is very hard to study the capacity of motor short-term memory when the number of motor items presented to a subject is not easily controlled.

One study that attempted to overcome this shortcoming in the motor short-term memory literature was by Wilberg and Salmela (1973). They used a two-dimensional joystick that could be moved in different directions with varying movement extents. With this apparatus the subjects were presented with a sequence of 2, 4, 6, or 8 movements and then had to reproduce them. In one condition the movements were presented to the subjects by having them watch the presentation of slides on a wall in front of them. Each slide contained a circular visual field, representing the area of movement of the joystick, and the subject was told to move the joystick to a position indicated by a black dot that appeared in the circle. Thus, by presenting 2, 4, 6, or 8 slides, the experimenter could have the subject make the required number of movements. After they were made, the subject then had to attempt to reproduce them without looking at the joystick, which was positioned at chair height on his right side. In the other condition of interest the required number of movements was randomly generated by the subject himself, after which he attempted to reproduce them.

The results showed that when the subjects generated the movements themselves, recall of these movements was almost uninfluenced by the number of movements they had to reproduce. In other words, they reproduced 2 movements with the same accuracy as they reproduced 8 movements, which would indicate that a capacity had not been reached. However, when they had to move in relation to the presented slides, errors in reproduction got progressively larger as the number of movements increased.

Wilberg and Salmela interpreted these findings as indicating a capacity for motor short-term memory when the input (that is, proprioceptive feedback entering short-term memory) was from the visually presented positions. They reasoned that this type of input was unpredictable, and therefore carried a large information load that exceeded the capacity of short-term memory. To explain why a capacity was not evident for the subject-generated movements, they postulated that the subjects used motor plans or efference to base their movement reproductions on. Since these were initially produced by the performer, they were predictable and hence carried less information than the other class of movements. The only thing wrong with this latter interpretation is that subjects need not have based their reproductions on motor plans but rather could have used visualized or imagined locations. Thus, they could have visualized the sequence of movements they were going to make before they started to move and then simply based their reproductions on this information rather than motor plans. This interpretation is supported by the fact that 8 visual items would probably be within the immediate memory span. Wilberg and Salmela's study is valuable, however, in that it does demonstrate that for certain types of movements there appears to be a definite capacity to how much information can be stored concerning the sequence of producing movements.

Rate of Loss of Information from Short-Term Memory

Previously, short-term memory was defined as a system that loses information in the absence of sustained attention. In essence, this means that this storage system is an unstable one and if some or all of an individual's information processing capacity (attention) is not involved with the to-be-remembered information, it will be forgotten. Forgetting in short-term memory that is due to a lack of attention is best demonstrated by requiring a subject, after he is presented with the to-be-remembered information, to perform an attention-demanding task during the retention interval that is as unrelated as possible to the stored information. This procedure thus minimizes structural interference effects and assures that the subject cannot rehearse or think about the information he has to recall at the end of the retention interval. As will be seen from the following discussion, when this procedure is followed, considerable forgetting does occur, and thus a further limitation of short-term memory is demonstrated.

Nonmotor information. Perhaps the best example of forgetting in short-term memory due to a lack of attention is illustrated through the common everyday experience of attempting to retain an unfamiliar telephone number from the time it is located in a telephone book to the time when dialing is first begun. If during this short interval, an individual's attention is diverted from rehearsing the number by something like fumbling with the telephone book, there is a good possibility that part of the number will be forgotten.

Peterson and Peterson (1959) provide good experimental evidence to support the above subjective example. They required their subjects to recall single trigrams (such as, X-J-R) after retention intervals that varied from 3 to 18 seconds. During these retention intervals the subjects were required to count backwards by 3s or 4s from a three-digit number presented one second after the trigram. The results showed that subjects got progressively worse over the 18-second retention interval, as indicated by a drop from an average of 80 percent completely correct recall of the trigram at 3 seconds to only about an average of 10 percent completely correct recall at 18 seconds. Thus it would appear that this type of information is lost very rapidly in the absence of sustained attention.

The above study only had subjects retain a single trigram, and this may be considered not to be a very realistic task in terms of real-life situations. Usually, an individual is concerned with remembering much more complex information, and hence it would be informative to know what happens to the rate of loss of information for this type of information. Melton (1963) provides evidence that the greater the amount of information in short-term memory or, in other words, the closer the information comes to the capacity of short-term memory, the greater the possibility is of an error occurring in recall. By having subjects recall 1, 2, 3, 4, or 5 consonants over retention intervals varying from 4 to 32 seconds, he showed that the amount of forgetting in recall was a direct function of not only the length of the retention interval but also of the number of items to be recalled. In discussing these results along with other data, Melton points out that it appears as if it is the number of chunks of information that is the critical factor that determines the amount of forgetting rather than the number of actual items or elements in the to-be-remembered material. Thus 5 items that can be remembered as one chunk will be recalled with much greater accuracy than 5 items that cannot be put into a meaningful structure.

Motor information. The loss of information from motor short-term memory reveals somewhat of a different picture than that of nonmotor information. Some studies (Posner and Konick, 1966; Posner, 1967), have shown that occupying a subject's limited processing capacity during a retention interval failed to show any difference in the reproduction of a blind movement when compared to that of subjects who were allowed to just sit and rest during the retention interval. Surprisingly, both of these conditions showed that subjects became worse in their reproductions over the retention interval. This finding has been interpreted as meaning that movement per se cannot be represented in short-term memory in a manner that allows it to be mentally rehearsed. Because of this, it is thought that whatever constitutes the representation of a pure motor act (that is, some form of a memory trace) starts to lose its information immediately after it enters the short-term memory system.

However, these results must be interpreted cautiously because, first, the area of investigation concerned with motor short-term memory is still in its infancy, and there are not many studies that have actually dealt with this problem and, second, as mentioned previously, the type of movement used in these studies is a rather unrealistic simple movement that may not represent the movements performed in everyday situations. Related to this latter point is the fact that there is not much known about what type of information an individual uses when attempting to reproduce a movement. Most studies have denied vision to their subjects, and therefore the major source of information presumably should be proprioceptive in nature. Usually, the standard or criterion movement is presented to a blindfolded subject by having him move his arm a certain distance by moving a cursor along a linear, almost frictionless track. He then has to return his arm to a starting position and, after the appropriate retention interval, attempt to reproduce the criterion movement as accurately as possible by again moving the cursor to where he thinks the end position of the movement is. Supposedly, since the subject is blindfolded and the cursor is either silent or the subject wears earmuffs to mask the noise of the cursor, the subject makes his reproduction in light of the proprioceptive information received while he performed the criterion movement. To maximize the possibility that subjects will have only proprioceptive information available on which to base their reproduction, the experimenter must be very careful to control for vision and audition since these variables can influence movement reproduction. The subject should not be allowed to see the movement apparatus before he is tested since this could give him a visual image to which he can relate the proprioceptive information received while being tested. Unfortunately, even this procedure does not guarantee that the subject will not use some form of visual imagery to aid his movement reproduction. The importance of vision in the learning of movement will be discussed in a later section of this book.

Even in those studies that minimize the possibility that their subjects will use some form of visual guidance, there still is a problem of determining what type of information is used by a subject. A number of recent studies (Keele and Ells, 1972; Laabs, 1973; Marteniuk and Roy, 1972; Marteniuk, 1973) have been concerned with isolating different proprioceptive cues upon which movement reproduction is based. The necessity for this type of investigation is realized when one contemplates the large range of information about a movement that might be stored in short-term memory. Information about the rate, time, and direction of the movement are all that a subject theoretically needs for reproduction of that movement. Yet other factors like the muscular effort required or the pattern of motor commands to the muscle might also be retained for use at a later time. Two other cues that would appear to be important in movement reproduction are information about movement extent and location.

In this respect, Marteniuk and Roy (1972) have shown that distance or extent cues were not as reliable as location cues in that subjects forced to use distance information could not reproduce a movement as well as subjects using only location cues. However, this study only dealt with reproduction after no delay interval, and therefore nothing can be said about the rate of loss of this information. Laabs (1973) did include retention intervals when he studied how well location and distance cues were retained. His results proved most interesting in that distance information became less exact over a 12-second retention interval regardless of whether the subjects just rested during this time or had their limited information processing capacity occupied by counting backwards. Of most interest, however, was the finding for subjects who were required to reproduce only location information. Here, when subjects counted backwards during the 12-second retention interval they became less accurate in their recall scores than the subjects in the distance condition. But when the location condition subjects were allowed to rest and think about the movement during the retention interval there was no loss of information in that movement reproduction was just as accurate as in the immediate reproduction group.

What these results seem to be implying is that some proprioceptive information is capable of entering short-term memory and being represented in such a manner that it allows an individual somehow to mentally rehearse the information so that it is not forgotten over a relatively short retention interval. Laabs (1973) suggests that perhaps there are two types of motor short-term memory. One is a central type of memory, wherein proprioceptive information can be coded and rehearsed in a manner analogous to what happens when people code and rehearse verbal or visual material. On the other hand, there appears to be another short-term storage system in which certain types of proprioceptive information are lost automatically or spontaneously over time.

The central type of memory system that was postulated by Laabs (1973) is called "central" because it is envisaged as having access to the limited central processing capacity of an individual. Here, as was explained in Chapter 3, central processing capacity is equated with the concept of attention. Thus, just as the retention of visual information has been shown to be aided by the presence of central processing capacity, it is likewise suggested that the retention of some aspects of motor information may also rely on this variable. From this viewpoint, one might say that an individual is capable of rehearsing proprioceptive or motor information (Marteniuk, 1973) and that this rehearsal is seen as affecting the retention of motor information in a manner similar to what occurs with repeated trials on a movement reproduction task; that is, repetition or physical practice has been shown to increase the accuracy of motor performance (Adams and Dijkstra, 1966; Stelmach and Bassin, 1971).

Interference in Motor Short-Term Memory

At the beginning of this section on short-term memory two types of interference that led to forgetting of information in short-term memory were described. It was pointed out that the specific cause of interference was determined by whether an attention-demanding interpolated task, performed during the retention interval of a short-term memory experiment, was either related or unrelated to the psychological structure of the to-be-remembered information. If the interpolated task was unrelated, interference was seen as being caused by the fact that the task was attention-demanding, and as a result prevented rehearsal of the information already in short-term memory. On the other hand, if a related interpolated task was used, this was seen as not only preventing rehearsal but also interfering with the psychological structure of the to-be-remembered material.

In the immediately preceding section, dealing with the rate of loss of information from motor short-term memory, it was seen that several studies (Marteniuk and Roy, 1972; Laabs, 1973; and Marteniuk, 1973) indicated that an unrelated attention-demanding interpolated task caused significant forgetting of movement information. This, thus, would indicate that at least some type of movement information require some or all of the limited information processing capacity if the information is to be retained. This finding has a number of implications for both the researcher and teacher of perceptual-motor skills. The practical implications will be presented in the next section of this chapter, and the research implications will be developed in Chapter 7.

The study of interference in motor short-term memory of the structural type has been investigated using two types of experimental paradigms. One paradigm, used to study *retroactive* interference, is exactly the same as has been described previously in this chapter. That is, the potentially interfering activity is performed after presentation of the criterion movement to determine whether it will retroactively interfere with the psychological structure of the criterion movement. The other paradigm is designed to investigate *proactive* interference. Here the potentially interfering activity is performed before the criterion movement is presented. The criterion is then performed and recall of this criterion is usually required immediately afterward. Thus, if interference occurs in this situation it is caused by information presented prior to the criterion movement.

In terms of the research evidence as to whether movement information in short-term memory can be structurally interfered with, conflicting results have been obtained. Stelmach (1974) presents an excellent review of much of this literature. His review shows that for the retroactive paradigm no interference occurs if the interpolated movement is similar to the criterion movement and is performed only once. However, if these interpolated movements are performed more than once, recall of the criterion movement is adversely influenced. For the effect that proactive interference has on information stored in motor short-term memory, Stelmach's (1974) review shows that the number of movements performed prior to the criterion movement being presented is also a crucial variable. If subjects are required to make several movements that are unrelated to the criterion movement and before they make the criterion movement, their recall of the criterion is less accurate than that of subjects who did not make the initial movements. Thus physical activity done prior to learning a movement seems to interfere with the short-term retention of that movement.

Although the above discussion serves as a short overview of work on interference in motor short-term memory, the reader should be aware of two shortcomings of this area of research. First, there are relatively few studies completed that deal specifically with motor interference, and thus no extensive findings or concrete conclusions can be reported at this time. Second, none of the work to date has been able to explain how motor interference occurs, just that it does. What is needed is more information on the psychological structure that motor information takes in short-term memory so that more precise predictions can be made as to exactly why physical activity interferes with the stored information. This not only would facilitate the theoretical development of motor short-term memory but it also would be of considerable benefit to understanding how this system operates in the performance and learning of perceptual-motor skills.

Facilitating Retention of Information in Short-Term Memory

From the above discussion on the capacity and retention characteristics of short-term information memory a number of implications can be derived concerning those factors leading to improved retention of information in short-term memory. These factors, since they can be under the control of a teacher or coach of perceptual-motor skills, are of considerable importance since storage of information in memory is an integral part of the instruction process. Basically, the two main headings under which these factors can be grouped are coding of information and rehearsal.

Although coding of motor information in short-term memory will be discussed in considerable detail in a later chapter in respect to the topic of learning, it now will be of interest to consider it under the topic of what Miller (1956) refers to as chunking. As was mentioned previously, this is the process whereby an individual groups together a number of items entering short-term memory into meaningful units. By this procedure an individual whose short-term memory capacity is about seven items can retain a large number of items by grouping them into chunks of information so that the number of chunks, rather than the number of individual items, determines the capacity of this memory system. An example of using chunking to help facilitate the retention of information occurs in the instruction process. Suppose that a teacher is describing the overhead clear in badminton to a group of students. Obviously there are many individual components or items that are of importance in the execution of this skill, and, of importance here, taken as a whole the number of items probably exceeds the capacity of the novice performer's ability to retain information. For instance, the main components of the overhead clear are the grip, stance, backswing, forward swing, point of contact with the shuttlecock, and the follow-through. Each one of these components, in turn, is composed of several smaller components. Thus, if a teacher attempts to describe the whole skill in detail, chances are that a good deal of the description will be lost. A wise teacher might want to simplify the skill by chunking a good deal of the components of the skill into meaningful units. One way this can be done is by describing to the students how the action of the overhead clear is similar to throwing a ball. Since most people have had experience in throwing, this immediately allows them to think of the badminton skill in terms of an already established experience, which in turn would allow them to remember the clear under the label "ball throw." In effect, a large number of items have been chunked under one label. Another label that produces the same result can be applied to the description of the racket at the end of the backswing. Here, the position of the elbow, the action of the wrist and the location of the racket can be chunked under the description "back-scratching position." A teacher, then, instead of sending his pupils out to practice some large number of items, might start out by telling them that while they are practicing they should keep in mind the actions involved in "throwing a ball" and in "back scratching." Obviously, other descriptive and familiar terms can be used to help "code" other individual items in the clear, so that a performer might have four or five pieces of information that contain all the necessary information required to perform the skill.

In essence, this chunking of information reduces the total uncertainty to a performer and allows him to deal with information loads within his capacity. The success of this technique is probably limited only by the ability of the teacher to group components of a skill successfully into meaningful units that allow for easy labeling and retention by his pupils.

The second way in which the retention of information in short-term memory can be facilitated is through rehearsal or, in other words, by attending to the information stored in this system. Figure 15 depicts this process, and implies that information is "strengthened" when an individual thinks about or attends to it. The relationship between short-term memory and attention, as depicted by the arrows, is analogous to a feedback loop indicating a repetition effect for every cycle, where repetition in

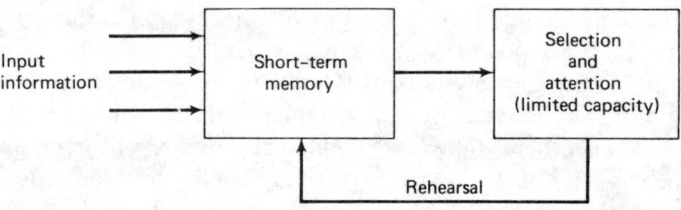

FIGURE 15   Facilitating short-term memory through selection of an attention to information.

this case is simply covertly thinking about the information. The necessity for this type of process is very evident for visual and auditory information and, while not so clear for motor information, evidence does seem to suggest that spatial or location information can be rehearsed in this manner.

Just as important as the fact that retention of information in short-term memory can be facilitated by attending to it is the consideration that information, both motor and nonmotor, is lost rapidly in the absence of sustained attention. In other words, if attention is focused elsewhere, thus interrupting the loop between short-term memory and attention in Figure 15, stored information is forgotten quickly. This certainly has implications for instruction purposes by implying that new information must be, at least initially, continually attended to so that its chances of being retained are increased. This means that a teacher not only must reduce or eliminate attention-demanding distractions in the instruction situation but also must get his students to attend to the new material either overtly or covertly.

Overt attention, of course, is best demonstrated either by having an individual physically practice a skill or by having him verbally explain the requirements of the skill just after the teacher has finished describing it. One way a teacher can have all individuals within a group think about the material just presented is to announce that, for the sake of review, one student will have to summarize the description of the new skill. If the teacher pauses for a short time after this statement, during which time everyone in the group should be mentally preparing himself for a presentation, then names the individual he wants the summary from, chances are that most students will have at least attempted to rehearse the new information. If a teacher uses this technique from day to day, it will also facilitate attention during his presentation since the students will come to know that any one of them might be required to give the summary description.

Finally, even though a teacher can control the attention of his students for short periods of time, chances are that during the interval between descriptions of the skill and the actual physical performance of it, there will arise many attention-distracting situations. In this case, then, since information is lost rapidly from short-term memory, the time interval between presentation of a description and performance of the new skill is crucial. A teacher should attempt to minimize this interval and get his students practicing the skill as soon as possible. Of course, related to this attempt at controlling the interval between presentation of new material and performance is the controlling of physical activity that could structurally interfere with the psychological form of the new activity in the performer's short-term memory. Here considerations of how proactive and retroactive interference might affect the retention of a new skill must be provided for in the daily lesson plan of the teacher.

Anticipation in Perceptual Motor Performance

As discussed previously under the topic of selective attention, the ability to anticipate the occurrence of proprioceptive feedback is an important feature of highly skilled performance. Anticipation, as was pointed out, effectively reduces the amount of information a performer has to process, which in turn reduces the complexity of monitoring the feedback occurring from the execution of the skill. The purpose of this present section is to discuss other types of anticipation that occur in perceptual motor behavior and to identify some of the factors that contribute to this ability.

Anticipation is necessary in the performance of perceptual-motor skills because of the delay that occurs between the occurrence of some event and an individual's initiation of a movement in response to that event. This interval of time, called reaction time, is an inevitable aspect of all performance. If performance in some skill can be seen as involving a series of reactions to varying environmental demands, and if each reaction involved about 200 milliseconds, performance should be characterized by a series of spasmodic movements, with a 200-millisecond delay between each movement. The fact that skilled performers do not move in this way, but usually exhibit smooth, continuous movements that constantly meet the demands of the environment, suggest that the basic delay of the reaction time is somehow compensated for.

It is proposed that the way performers overcome this delay is through anticipation, and this process can best be understood in terms of Norman's (1969) model of selective attention (Figure 14). In particular, the part of the model that explains anticipation in perceptual-motor skills is the component dealing with past experience and contextual cues. This model implies that through learning a performer builds up a vast reservoir of experience that he can use to interpret the events encountered in situations similar to previously experienced situations. In essence, a performer through the use of past experience makes "best-bet" judgments as to what will likely happen in a given situation. This type of anticipation allows an individual to begin responding before the onset of a particular event, which thus leaves time for the delay due to his reaction time.

In the language of information processing it can be said that a performer is taking advantage of the redundancy in perceptual-motor skills to allow him to circumvent the basic limitation imposed on him by the delay due to reaction time. Redundancy, in this sense, implies a reduction of information due to the fact that through past experience a performer can predict what will happen in a sequence of events because the first part of the sequence signals or implies the occurrence of the later parts. This type of prediction or anticipation takes many forms in perceptual-motor skills and it will be beneficial at this point to consider two such examples.

Anticipation in Hitting or Catching a Ball

In many skills there is a necessity to hit or catch a ball that sometimes travels over 100 miles per hour. If it takes 200 milliseconds for a performer to react to an event, this must mean that his decision to react must be made while the ball is a considerable distance from him because in 200 milliseconds a ball traveling at 100 miles per hour can cover a large distance. Also, since reaction time does not take into account movement time (the time it takes the performer to move his body or limbs to hit or catch the ball), the decision to react must be made when the ball is even farther away from him.

One study (Scott, 1945) demonstrated that a baseball thrown overhand can travel a distance of 60½ feet (the distance from the rubber on the pitcher's mound to home plate) in a time of 430 to 580 milliseconds. As Whiting (1969) points out, if it is assumed that a visual reaction time is involved, this means that on the average a player would have to initiate his swing when the ball was about 25 feet away. Further, since these figures do not take into account movement time, the initiation of the swing would probably have to take place even further back in time. However, it may be that baseball players initiate a general swing on every pitch so that movement is under way before they react to the specific characteristics of the pitched ball. If this is the case, the decision to carry through with the swing or hold it back might have to be made when the ball is only about 25 feet away.

How is it then that batters—and in a similar way, catchers—usually enjoy a fair amount of success? Obviously what is required is some type of anticipation that allows them to predict where the ball will be when, in the case of the batter, it crosses home plate, or for the catcher, it approaches his hands so it can be caught. This means that the performer must be able to interpret cues from the ball, early in its flight, that predict where the ball will be as it nears him. This prediction ability is a function of learning, and the more experience a performer has in catching or hitting balls, the better he will be at making these types of predictions. For the batter, additional cues about where the ball will be thrown might come from certain idiosyncrasies of the pitcher that signal what type of pitch will be thrown. From this information plus the information gained from the ball's early flight path, the batter might be able to predict quite accurately where the ball will cross the plate. Similarly, an individual catching a ball not only has information from the flight of the ball but also might be able to gain some information from the source the ball was delivered from. If a ball is thrown, the catcher can see the action of the thrower and make a prediction about the speed and direction of the throw.

Anticipating Proprioceptive Feedback

Proprioceptive feedback was discussed in the section on selective attention and therefore will not be treated in any detail here. The particular behavior of interest is the ability of highly skilled players to anticipate what the characteristics of the proprioceptive feedback will be that they receive from executing a particular movement. This ability is important for two reasons. First, it reduces the amount of information that a performer has to monitor in that his anticipated feedback is based on what he intended to do. Thus if he actually executes the skill as intended, the ensuing feedback is redundant, since it was predicted or anticipated, and as a result monitoring the feedback takes very little of the performer's central processing capacity. Second, anticipating feedback is important for error correction purposes. Since proprioceptive feedback occurs in advance of knowledge about what the result of movement execution is (that is, where the ball went after it was hit), it can be used to correct late components of the movement, provided that the movement is not so rapid that there is no time to process feedback. Error correction here would be seen as involving a comparison between anticipated feedback and the feedback received from the proprioceptive receptors activated by the movement.

The above uses of anticipated feedback obviously are possible only in highly skilled performers. At the base of this ability is, again, a collection of past experiences that allow a performer to predict the sequence of proprioceptive signals that he will receive while executing a skill. This is another example of how a performer can take advantage of redundancy in perceptual motor skills.

In way of summary of the above two examples, and again to emphasize what anticipation involves, it is worthwhile to reconsider Norman's model of selective attention, presented in Figure 14. His main point is that processing of perceptual information is tremendously aided by a performer's expectations. These expectations are a result of learning the sequential dependencies present in the information of interest. Norman (1969) uses the skill of reading to explain this process in that an average reader can process between 300 to 600 words each minute, and this implies that he must identify as many as 10 words or 50 to 70 letters per second. Since this is faster than the recognition process is capable of operating, the reader must be making use of the constraints within a grammatical text. In other words, the English language is highly redundant (about 50 percent in fact) in that there are: (1) relatively few sequences of letters that can appear within a word; (2) relatively few sequences of words that can occur in a meaningful sentence; and (3) relatively few sequences of ideas that can logically appear on a page of written material. Thus the reader, in taking advantage of these constraints needs only a little information from individual letters or words and can probably skip many of them without losing the content of the message of any given page of text.

It is argued that just like in reading a page of grammatical text, a skilled perceptual motor performer becomes very adept at determining the dependencies that exist in these skills and makes use of them in the perceptual recognition process. This process is the basis for anticipation, and without this ability a performer would not be able to cope successfully with the demands required for highly skilled performance.

Anticipation and Timing of Movements

The above discussion of anticipation was based mostly on the ability of a performer to predict, from an early component in a sequence of events, the end result of that sequence. It was mentioned that this anticipation was necessary because, without it, the delay in performance imposed by a performers reaction time would severely handicap him in meeting the demands of fast perceptual motor skills. Implied in this description of anticipation was the ability of the performer, upon knowing or predicting a sequence of events, to coincide his response with the demands of the environment. This aspect of performance will be called coincidence timing. Poulton (1957) has described three forms of this type of anticipation, and these are discussed below.

Effector Anticipation

Effector anticipation involves predicting or anticipating only the time a movement will take. This type of time prediction is necessary whenever a performer's movement must coincide with some external environmental demand, such as a ball in flight. A batter, conceivably, could be able to read a pitched ball very accurately and know what type of swing to perform, but if he is unable to time the duration of his swing so that his bat coincides with the ball as it crosses the plate his performance will not be successful.

Receptor Anticipation

Poulton (1957) describes receptor anticipation as involving the ability to predict the duration of some external event like a pitched ball. Thus a batter must know not only where the ball will cross the plate but also when it will arrive. Receptor anticipation also implies effector anticipation in that the performer must predict the duration of his response so that it coincides with the anticipated time of arrival of the external event.

Perceptual Anticipation

Perceptual anticipation is the most complex, in that it involves the anticipation of time in a sequence of movements where there is no direct receptor anticipation of these events. A good example of this type of timing is a gymnast performing a sequence of movements on some apparatus. Timing is an important aspect of this performance in that each component of his routine must be initiated at the exact moment of completion of the previous component. Thus he must be concerned with ordering the components of his skill and also the timing of this ordering. One way that such timing might be learned is through the use of proprioceptive feedback. Earlier it was explained how the anticipation of this feedback helped reduce the information load in monitoring the execution of a skill as well as how it played a role in movement error correction. In the present context, it may also be implicated in timing a sequence of events in that certain aspects of feedback from the initial component of a routine may be used as a stimulus to initiate the second component; in turn, certain aspects of feedback from the second component could lead to initiation of the third component, and so on.

Summary

This chapter has attempted to explain in some detail those perceptual processes that limit the pickup of information by the human performer. The perceptual mechanism is the first information processing step in the chain of processes that eventually transform an input into a movement. A major emphasis in this chapter was to demonstrate, in many cases, where those perceptual processes that underlie the processing of verbal and visual information are no different from those contributing to successful perceptual-motor performance. Thus, in being consistent with the theme of the book, we have seen where a good part of perceptual-motor skills, oftentimes referred to as "motor" skills, are in reality highly cognitive in nature and require very complex psychological processes.

Another emphasis in the chapter, and again one that is consistent with the theme of this book, was that many of the perceptual information processes that contribute to perceptual-motor skills also are important in successful teaching, which we considered a communication skill. This was especially apparent in the treatment of selective attention and short-term memory, where these processes were seen to be important in receiving and retaining information both from an environment in which an individual is performing some perceptual-motor skill and from an environment in which an individual is listening to the instructions of a teacher.

Another common theme of this chapter was the way in which many of the processes limited a performer's ability to sense, attend to, recognize, and retain perceptual information. Sensory abilities, while not being that important for the performance of perceptual-motor skills, were considered to be important in that the study of the properties of sensory systems can lead to valuable knowledge about how information sensed by them is used in the performance and learning of skills. Signal detection theory, on the other hand, was seen to be valuable for recognizing how performers make rapid decisions in fast-moving games and while under the influence of stress.

Selective attention and short-term memory were two processes that seemed to place the largest limitations on the perceptual mechanism in terms of its ability to process information. It was shown how a performer can attend only to a limited source of information and how he can retain only about seven items in memory. However, upon closer study of these processes, it was shown that in many cases their limitations can be overcome if the performer makes use of redundant information and recodes information into chunks to facilitate its retention.

Finally, the role of anticipation in perceptual-motor performance was discussed in a separate section. Anticipation was seen as basically a perceptual process, and was explained by the utilization of past experience by an individual to interpret environmental and proprioceptive information. A number of different types of anticipation were defined, and the role that this ability plays in perceptual-motor skills was explained.

Suggested Readings

Signal Detection Theory

McNicol, D., *A Primer of Signal Detection Theory.* London: G. Allen, 1972.
Swets, J. A., *Signal Detection and Recognition by Human Observers.* New York: Wiley, 1964.
Welford, A. T., *Fundamentals of Skill*, London: Methuen, 1968.

Information Comparison

Alphern, M., Lawrence, M., and Wolsk, D., *Sensory Processes.* Belmont, Calif.: Brooks/Cole, 1967.
Welford, A. T., *Fundamentals of Skill.* London: Methuen, 1968.
Woodworth, R. S., and Schlosberg, H., *Experimental Psychology.* New York: Holt, Rinehart and Winston, 1954.

Absolute Judgment

Fitts, P. M., and Posner, M. I., *Human Performance*, Belmont, Calif.: Brooks/Cole, 1967.

Garner, W. R., An informational analysis of absolute judgments of loudness. *Journal of Experimental Psychology*, 1953, **46,** 373–380.

Garner, W. R., and Hake, H. W., Amount of information in absolute judgments. *Psychological Review*, 1951, **58,** 446–449.

Kinesthesis

Howard, I. P., and Templeton, W. B., *Human Spatial Orientation*. New York: Wiley, 1966.

Keele, S. W., Movement control in skilled motor performance. *Psychological Bulletin*, 1968, **70,** 387–403.

Marteniuk, R. G., and Hayes, K., Kinesthetic information and the control of movement. In H. T. A. Whiting (Ed.), *Readings in Human Performance and Sports Psychology*. London: Lepus, 1975.

Smith, Judith L., Kinesthesis: A model for movement feedback. In R. C. Brown, Jr. and B. J. Cratty (Ed.), *New Perspectives of Man in Action*, Englewood Cliffs, N. J.: Prentice-Hall, 1969.

Williams, Harriet G., Neurological concepts and perceptual-motor behavior. In R. C. Brown, Jr. and B. J. Cratty (Ed.), *New Perspectives of Man in Action*, Englewood Cliffs, N. J.: Prentice-Hall, 1969.

Selective Attention

Keele, S. W., *Attention and Human Performance*. Pacific Palisades, Calif.: Goodyear, 1973.

Lindsay, P. H., and Norman, D. A., *Human Information Processing*. New York: Academic Press, 1972.

Norman, D. A., *Memory and Attention*, New York: Wiley, 1969.

Short-Term Memory

Fitts, P. M., and Posner, M. I., *Human Performance*. Belmont, Calif.: Brooks/Cole, 1967.

Posner, M. I., Short term memory systems in human information processing. *Information-Processing Approaches to Visual Perceptions*. New York: Holt, Rinehart and Winston, 1969.

Stelmach, G. E., Retention of motor skills. In J. T. Wilmore (Ed.), *Exercise and Sport Sciences Reviews*. New York: Academic Press, 1974.

Anticipation in Perceptual Motor Performance

Poulton, E. C., On prediction in skilled movement. *Psychological Bulletin,* 1957.

Schmidt, R. A., Anticipation and timing in human motor performance. *Psychological Bulletin*, 1968, **70,** 631–646.

Whiting, H. T. A., *Acquiring Ball Skill, A Psychological Interpretation.* Philadelphia: Lea & Febiger, 1969.

Chapter 5

The Decision Mechanism

The previous chapter discussed some of the factors within the perceptual mechanism that limited the amount of information able to be processed by a performer. In general it was found that a considerable compression of input information occurred, with perceptual identification and classification being based on relatively small amounts of information when compared to the large amounts present in the environment or in the proprioceptive feedback from a response. As was discussed earlier, however, the result of information processing within the perceptual mechanism is a perceptual response, which represents what has been perceived, that is sent to the decision mechanism. In terms of the model presented in Figure 2, Chapter 1, the decision mechanism then must, in the light of current objectives, decide upon a plan of action. Accordingly, the purpose of this chapter will be to discuss what limitations are imposed on a performer in terms of his ability to choose a plan of action. Again, as in the perceptual mechanism, this analysis will mostly take the form of limitations in information processing ability.

Reaction Time as a Measure of Decision Time

Ever since psychologists first became interested in determining the speed with which people could make decisions, the topic of reaction time has always received considerable attention. Reaction time has come to be defined as the delay occurring between the presentation of some event or stimulus to an individual and the *initiation* of movement to that stimulus. The phrase "initiation of movement" is used because theoretically reaction time only includes the time it takes: (1) for a stimulus to activate a particular sensory receptor; (2) for the resulting signal to travel to the brain; (3) for the signal to be processed by the brain; and (4) for a command to be sent down from the brain to some muscle or group of muscles. Thus reaction time does not include any muscular contraction time. However, for convenience of measurement, usually very small movements like a finger press or release are used with the assumption that the movement time or delay for very simple movements is insignificant when compared to the size of the delay due to the previously listed factors.

Helmholtz in the 1850s contributed significantly to the concept of reaction time when he determined the approximate speed of the nerve transmission time to and from the brain. Up to this time there was no real evidence to indicate just what caused the delay in reaction time in that it could be caused by slow peripheral nerve transmission time and/or slow processing in the brain. To determine the delay in peripheral nerve transmission time Helmholtz stimulated a subject on the thigh and on the sole of the foot and determined the difference between these two reaction times. Since the two stimuli were the same, he reasoned that any difference between the two reaction times must be due to the extra nerve conduction length that the stimulation from the sole of the foot had to travel. On the basis of this difference between the two reaction times he concluded the neural impulses travel at the rate of 50 to 100 meters per second. Since Helmholtz's time these figures have been generally upheld, and therefore from this type of work one can readily determine that peripheral nerve conduction time per se would account for only a very small portion of reaction time. Since simple visual and auditory reaction times (by simple is meant that there is only one fixed stimulus) usually range between about 150 to 200 milliseconds, it can be concluded that most of this delay must occur in the brain itself.

The question of interest, then, is: What are the factors that produce the delay in performance due to reaction time? It can be assumed that factors that cause relatively large delays would impair perceptual-motor performance where speed or quickness of response was an important component of the performance. In this way the decision process can be seen as limiting the ability of an individual to rapidly process information about the requirement of a skill. Before discussing the sources or causes of these delays, it is necessary to talk briefly about the measurement of information. Since the ability to process information rapidly is an important characteristic of perceptual-motor skills, being able to measure how much information can be processed per unit of time will be a valuable aid in quantifying the capacity of an individual to make decisions.

Measurement of Information

One way of conceptualizing the decision processes involved in perceptual motor skills is to compare this process to a channel in which input information must be analyzed. If the channel is very large, obviously a lot of information can pass through it very quickly, and decision times would be relatively fast. On the other hand, if the channel were small, only small amounts of information could be processed per unit time, and if a response was contingent on processing large amounts of information, the processing time would be relatively long. Thus, two aspects of information processing in the above context become important when attempting to study decision processes in perceptual motor skills. First, what is the size of the channel through which information can be processed? Second, if the size of the channel can be specified, how can the *amount* of input information be quantified?

The size of the channel and quantifying the amount of input information to it are important considerations for various reasons. One reason is that it has been thought (Welford, 1960) that the decision process has a definite channel capacity in that only so much information can be processed per unit time. This channel capacity would explain why an individual, faced with a large amount of information, would take a long time to react. However, the concept of channel capacity by itself is insufficient to explain skilled performance, since a general characteristic of perceptual-motor skills is that an individual reacts quicker through practice or learning. This might possibly imply, from our channel analogy, that the channel is becoming larger through practice and as a result can process more information per unit time. On the other hand, another reason for the faster decision times, and one that has considerable power for understanding some of the processes underlying perceptual motor skills, is that through learning or practice the amount of input information for a given skill or game becomes less. As a result the skilled performer, with the same channel capacity as he had when he was a naive beginner, has much less information to process and therefore can decide upon a plan of action in a much shorter time.

From the above, then, it is assumed that a performer has a relatively fixed capacity to process information regarding decisions about selecting a plan of action. Speed of making decisions, however, is facilitated by reducing the amount of input information to the channel so that it takes a shorter time to arrive at a decision. In this light it will now be informative to examine more closely what is meant by amount of information and ways in which it is quantified. Once the reader understands how information is measured, the study of the factors in perceptual-motor skills that govern the amount of information with which a performer is faced can then be undertaken.

As mentioned and implied in previous chapters, the concept of the amount of information is exactly opposite to what one intuitively thinks it is. In terms of how it is used here, the amount of information is directly related to the amount of uncertainty presented to an individual. In perceptual motor skills there are many potential sources of uncertainty confronting a performer. Chief among these sources are the *number* of possible events or alternative plans of action confronting an individual, as well as their *predictability*. The larger the number of alternative events or the greater their unpredictability, the larger the amount of information confronting an individual. Similarly, as the number of events becomes fewer or as they become more predictable, the less the amount of information becomes. The extreme case, in which there would be no information present, would be where there is only one possible event and an individual knows exactly when and where it will occur.

One can now appreciate the task faced by a naive performer with a fixed channel capacity for deciding among alternative events. In a game situation, for example, the environment contains a great deal of uncertainty in that there are a great number of alternative events occurring and, moreover, the performer has no way of determining what events are most probable, given certain situations. Usually, because of this great uncertainty, performance is characterized by slow and/or inaccurate responses.

At the other extreme is the case of the highly skilled performer. Although the same channel capacity limitation holds, because of a great deal of experience he is faced with small amounts of information. Not only can the skilled performer dismiss many alternative courses of action as being highly improbable, but the remaining few can be ordered in terms of their probability of occurrence so that he is most ready for the most probable event. If he happens to be correct in his assignment of probabilities to events, which is a characteristic of highly skilled performers, there is very little uncertainty, and as a result his decision process is relatively simple and fast.

Experimentally, it is a relatively easy procedure to vary, separately or in combination, both the number of events an individual is presented with and the probability of occurrence of these events. To quantify the amount of information presented to a subject, the basic unit of measurement called a *bit* is used. The term "bit," an abbreviation of binary digit, is the amount of information needed to predict accurately which one of two equally likely events will occur. The number of bits of information is equivalent to the number of questions that must be asked to determine the correct alternative. For instance, if an individual has to make a decision between two equally likely alternative events he need only ask one question: is it event number 1? If the answer is yes, he has determined the correct alternative; if it is no, he has done the same thing because if it is not alternative one it must be alternative two. The amount of information conveyed by 8 equally probable alternative events is 3 bits. In essence, the correct choice was made by halving the alternatives three times until only the correct alternative is left. To illustrate, consider the problem of attempting to find what number a person is thinking of from the numbers 1 through 8. If three questions with yes-no answers are asked, the correct number can always be found. For instance, the first question might be whether the target number is in the first four numbers. If the answer is yes then the next question might be whether it is the first two numbers. If the answer is no the next question will allow discovery of the correct number.

Technically stated, the number of bits of information conveyed by any given number of events is:

$$\text{Bits} = \log_2 N$$

where N is the number of equally likely alternatives.

As was mentioned previously, a second way in which the amount of information conveyed by various events can vary is through the events having unequal probabilities. When a performer in a game situation knows that some events are much more probable than other events, there is a better chance of predicting what will happen. In this case the total number of events would carry less information than if they were all equally probable. When events are not equally probable, the formula for determining the amount of information conveyed by each event is:

$$\text{Bits} = \log_2 \frac{1}{p}$$

where p is the probability of that event occurring. To calculate the average amount of information that occurs in a sequence of events that might all have different probabilities of occurrence the following formula is used:

$$\text{Bits} = \sum_{i=1}^{N} p_i \log_2 \frac{1}{p_i}$$

The preceding two formulas reflect the fact that events that are very probable or sequences of events that tend always to occur in a particular order carry less information because of the reduction of their uncertainty. Certainly, in many perceptual-motor skills, especially of the open type, there is always a process whereby performers label some events as more probable than others or in which they come to know that certain acts or sets of cues tend to follow quite predictably from prior events. In this way the knowledgeable performer can considerably reduce the total amount of uncertainty faced by him.

Information and Decision Times

Temporal Uncertainty

In many open skills a major source of uncertainty facing the performer is concerned with his not knowing exactly when an event will occur. A good baseball pitcher will vary the speed of his pitched ball so that the batter will have some difficulty in predicting exactly when it will cross the plate. Likewise, an experienced tennis player will attempt to vary the speed of his returns in an effort to offset his opponent. In essence, the efforts of the pitcher or tennis player here are designed to keep his opponent from being able to anticipate, since, as was discussed in Chapter 4, anticipation is a very powerful device both for reducing the uncertainty of an event and for circumventing the delay associated with reaction time.

To demonstrate the effects of temporal uncertainty on reaction time Klemmer (1957) conducted a reaction time experiment. He reasoned that in an experimental situation there were two ways in which temporal uncertainty could be varied. The first source of uncertainty arises from the interval between a warning signal given to a subject and the actual presentation of the stimulus to respond; this period of time is called the foreperiod. The longer this foreperiod becomes, the more uncertainty there is because of a performer's inability to judge the passage of time accurately. The second source of uncertainty arises from the situation in which the length of the foreperiod is randomly varied. For example, foreperiods of 1, 2, 3, or 4 seconds might be used by an experimenter, and to avoid having the subject guess or anticipate what foreperiod will be used on any particular trial, the experimenter randomly orders their presentation. Thus anticipation is virtually impossible.

Klemmer (1957) thus varied the amount of information presented to his subjects, using calculations similar to those described earlier, so that at times there was very little uncertainty when the stimulus would be presented and at other times there was considerable uncertainty. His results indicated that as the number of bits of information due to temporal uncertainty was increased, his subjects' reaction times increased in a linear trend. The lowest amount of uncertainty resulted in a reaction time of about 150 milliseconds, whereas the greatest uncertainty produced a reaction time of approximately 250 milliseconds.

The only drawback in using Klemmer's results to generalize to situations occurring in open skills is the fact that in the experimental situation the stimulus suddenly appears after a given foreperiod, whereas in a sports skill situation the stimulus (for example, the ball or an opponent) is almost always in full view of the performer. Thus anticipation can occur much more readily in the real-life situation, and the effects of temporal uncertainty might tend to be minimized. Certainly, however, temporal uncertainty plays a large role in U.S. and Canadian football, where the quarterback varies the signal count for snapping the ball to keep the defense from anticipating. Also, any maneuver by a team or individual that tends to vary the pace of a game or speed of a ball would also be seen as an attempt to manipulate this variable.

Event Uncertainty (Choice Reaction Time)

As mentioned in the section on information measurement, there are three ways in which event uncertainty can influence the amount of information a performer is faced with: (1) As the number of events increase, amount of information increases; (2) as the probability of any given event increases, the amount of information conveyed by that event decreases; and, (3) if sequential dependencies are established among a group of events, the amount of information conveyed by the total number of events is reduced.

To determine how the number and probability of events influences reaction time the study of choice reaction time becomes necessary. Whereas simple reaction time involves a single stimulus and response, choice reaction time experiments involve more than one stimulus and more than one response. A typical way of investigating choice reaction time is through the use of an apparatus such as the one illustrated in Figure 16. If an investigator wishes to study event uncertainty he may wish to start by measuring simple reaction time which would represent the least amount of information and serve as a base line to compare choice reaction times to. Thus a subject might be given a number of trials on the apparatus in Figure 16 by having him place the index finger of his right hand (assuming that he is right-handed) on reaction key number 2 for the right hand. The signal for the subject to press the reaction key is the illumination of the light directly above key 2. Usually a random foreperiod between the warning light and stimulus light is utilized. Once an estimate of simple reaction time is obtained, the subject is then presented with a two-choice condition where he is asked to place his right and left index fingers on the

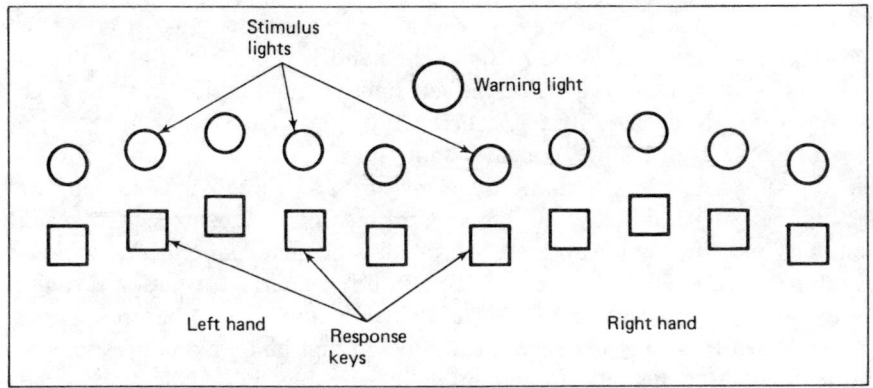

FIGURE 16   An example of a choice reaction time apparatus.

right and left number 2 keys, respectively. A series of trials is then presented where the probability of the occurrence of each stimulus (the light above the appropriate key) is equal. To avoid differences in reaction time due to the use of different fingers, the experimenter (unknown to the subject) just uses reaction times from the right index finger to calculate the time required to respond to two stimuli.

In a similar manner to the above, the experimenter can increase the number of stimuli and responses to 4, then 6, then 8, and finally 10, where all 8 fingers and 2 thumbs would be placed on the reaction keys. Usually, to avoid practice or familiarization effects, the subjects in a choice reaction time experiment would not normally take the various choice conditions in the order described above. Usually the conditions are randomly assigned to the different subjects, so each subject would perform the conditions in a different order.

Through the use of the same apparatus one can see how event probability and sequential dependencies can also be studied. Suppose, for example, that the ten-choice condition is used and that each subject is presented with 1000 trials. With so many trials it is possible for the experimenter to assign different probabilities of occurrence to each one of the stimuli. For instance, light number 2 of the right and left hand might both be presented 200 times during the course of the 1000 trials, which would make their probability of occurrence each .20. If the other eight lights were all presented an equal number of times (that is, 75 times each) their probability of occurrence would be .075. After the subject learned of these probabilities, which would not be too long, the influence of event uncertainty through different event probabilities could then be examined.

Sequential dependencies could also be established in a similar manner, except that in this case the experimenter introduces the probability of a given stimulus following the occurrence of another specific stimulus. It could be that whenever light number 2 of the right hand is presented, the probability of the corresponding light for the left hand occurring next is quite high compared to the probability of occurrence of any of the other lights.

The above discussion indicates that the amount of information contained in a set or series of stimuli can be varied in three ways: by varying the number of stimuli; by varying the probability of occurrence of each stimulus; and, by establishing sequential dependencies among the various stimuli. Hyman (1953), in a now classical study, varied information through the use of all these techniques. His choice reaction time apparatus was a little different from the one described above in that he had vocal responses, in the form of a name, to each of eight possible lights. He conducted three experiments, one for each of the techniques for varying amounts of information, and used four subjects, with each subject performing about 15,000 reaction times in more than 40 experimental sessions scheduled over a three-month period.

The results of Hyman's study proved to be remarkable in that for each of his four subjects reaction time was determined primarily by the amount of information represented by the specific conditions rather than by the manner in which information was varied. In other words, each experiment had amount of information varying from close to 0.0 bits to about 3.0 bits, and the subjects' reactions proved to be fastest at low levels of information and slowest at the highest levels. Moreover, the trend of reaction times over amount of information was very linear (correlations between reaction times and amount of information were well above .90) in nature for all three types of information, indicating the very powerful effect amount of information had on reaction time. Some idea of how amount of information affected reaction time can be seen by comparing reaction time at the two extremes of information. For 0 bits of information, reaction times for all four subjects tended to vary between about 160 to 200 milliseconds (this in essence was simple reaction time), whereas for information values close to 3.0 bits, reaction times varied from a little less than 600 milliseconds for one subject to a little more than 800 milliseconds for another subject. Further, since there was a linear relationship between amount of information and reaction time, Hyman determined that for each increase of information of one bit there was a constant increase of reaction time that varied from 127 to 215 milliseconds for his four subjects.

These results thus indicate that, regardless of how amount of information is manipulated, slow decision times can be expected when large amounts of information are present. The application to perceptual-motor skills, especially of the open type, seems to be direct since much of the information in the environment can be described by the number of events, event probabilities, or sequential dependencies among events. Highly skilled performers obviously take advantage of event probability and sequential dependencies, and by doing so they considerably reduce the amount of information and thus their decision times are considerably decreased. What these statements are implying is that to a considerable extent there is a great deal of redundancy in perceptual motor skills. Events, which can be taken as movements, ball flight, or patterns of movement, in team play tend to be highly structured. If a performer can learn this structure, he can take advantage of it and considerably reduce the demand on his information processing mechanisms. In effect, this section on event uncertainty is closely tied to some of the concepts on anticipation discussed in Chapter 4. The underlying principles are the same in that by reducing event uncertainty through knowledge about event probability or sequential dependencies, a performer is reducing the amount of information faced by him.

Perceptual Discrimination

The above discussion of event uncertainty was based on tasks in which the discriminability of the various events or signals was very clear. When this was the case, it was shown that as the number of events increased, reaction time became progressively slower. Now we consider the case where the degree of choice is held constant, but the discriminability among the choices is varied.

It has been known for some time that as signals come to resemble one another, the time taken to discriminate among them rises considerably. Henmon (1906), for instance, investigated this phenomenon by having his subjects attempt to discriminate rapidly which of two straight lines, exposed on a screen, was the shorter. The shorter line was always 10 centimeters in length, and the other line varied from 10.5 to 13.0 centimeters in 0.5 centimeter steps. Subjects signaled their response by pressing one of two reaction keys. Henmon's results indicated that the more the two lines came to resemble each other, the longer the reaction time.

In another experiment designed to investigate what effect discriminability had on decision time, Crossman (1955) required his subjects to sort specially prepared packs of cards into bins, depending on how many dots were on the card. Each card had small dots placed at random on its face and the number of dots could vary from one to twelve per card. In one part of his experiment Crossman had six decks of cards containing equal numbers of each of two different numbers of spots: 10 and 1; 10 and 5; 12 and 8; 12 and 9; 10 and 8; and 12 and 10. It can be seen that sorting a deck of cards with each card having either 10 random dots on its surface or just 1 dot would be much easier, from a perceptual discrimination viewpoint, than sorting a deck with cards containing either 12 or 10 dots.

Since sorting cards involves not only a decision time but also a considerable time due to the movement of placing a card in a given bin, Crossman also had his subjects sort the same number of blank cards into the bins. Since this latter condition had no decision time associated with it, it served as a control condition. The time to sort the blank cards was then subtracted from the time to sort the cards with dots, and the resulting difference represented decision time. The mean decision time per card could then be obtained by dividing the total decision time by the number of cards sorted. When this was done, and these mean times were plotted against the ratio of the dots on the cards (that is, 10/1, 10/5, 12/8, 12/9, 10/8, 12/10), it was found that discrimination time became slower as the ratio of the dots on the cards became smaller.

Both Henmon's and Crossman's data demonstrate that perceptual discrimination takes time, and the more difficult the discrimination the more time that is required. These results are almost identical to those discussed under event uncertainty, but in this case the uncertainty, or the information, arises from a perceptual source. However, the fact that a performer has a limited capacity to make decisions is again pointed out by the results, with the crucial factor determining this capacity being the amount of information that the performer has to process. An excellent review of this principle of human information processing, especially in regard to event and discrimination uncertainty can be found in an article by Welford (1960).

Perhaps the above results explain why some coaches of athletic skills stress the fact that their athletes should begin execution of a number of different movements in an identical manner. Take, for instance, the badminton player who is successful at initiating the overhead clear, drop, and smash in an identical fashion and it is not until late in the stroke that differentiating movements occur. In this case the opponent is faced not only with event uncertainty but also with uncertainty due to perceptual discrimination. The more closely an athlete can make different movements appear alike, the more time his opponent will have to spend in perceptually discriminating them.

The same principle occurs in U.S. and Canadian football, where a series of offensive plays is designed so that each play begins in an identical manner and it is not until quite late in the play's execution that it becomes apparent where the exact location of its point of attack will be. By designing a series of plays like this a coach is forcing the opposition to delay their decision until the last possible moment, when it might be too late to prevent the execution of the play.

Practice and Compatibility

The above discussions on temporal, event, and discrimination uncertainty have established that decision times become longer with increasing uncertainty. As pointed out by Fitts and Posner (1967), Welford (1968), and Keele (1973), the relationship between uncertainty (or, more specifically, amount of information) and decision time can be described by a linear trend, with fast times related to low amounts of information and slow times associated with high amounts of information. This type of relationship can be seen in the various lines of Figure 17. Although this figure is concerned primarily with event uncertainty, the same type of relationships exist for temporal and discrimination uncertainty.

Upon inspection of Figure 17 one thing becomes immediately apparent. The slopes of the lines are all different, with some slopes being almost flat. This latter fact would indicate that for some tasks the performer would seem to have an almost unlimited capacity to process information in that no matter how much information is present he processes it in the

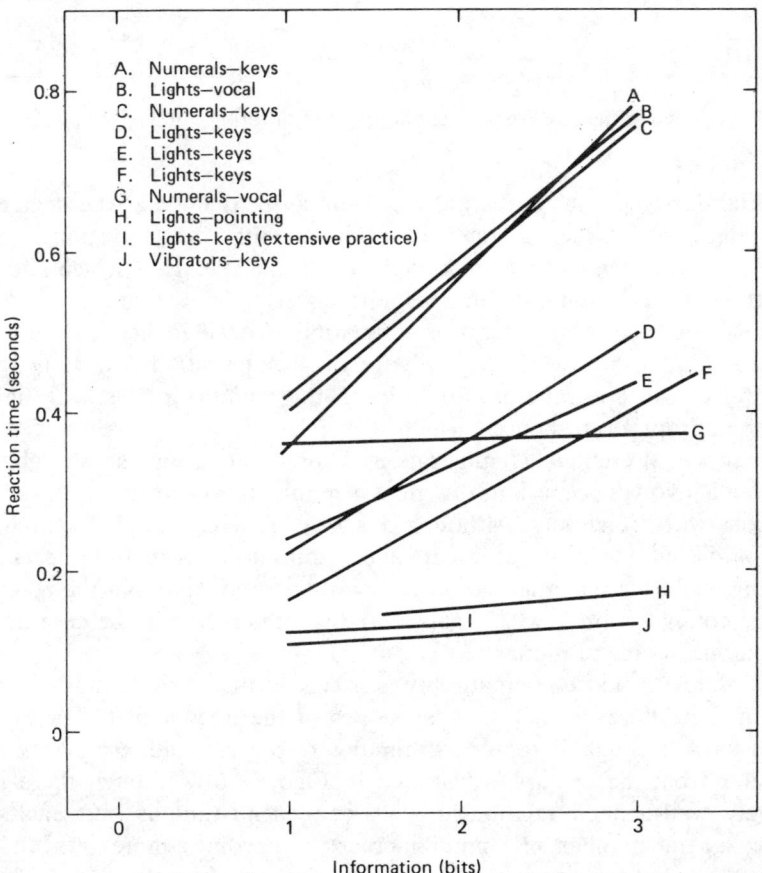

FIGURE 17 The effect of stimulus-response compatibility on decision times (from Fitts and Posner (1967).

same amount of time. Why is it, then, that some tasks seem not to be influenced by the amount of information to be processed? The reasons are twofold; stimulus-response compatibility and practice.

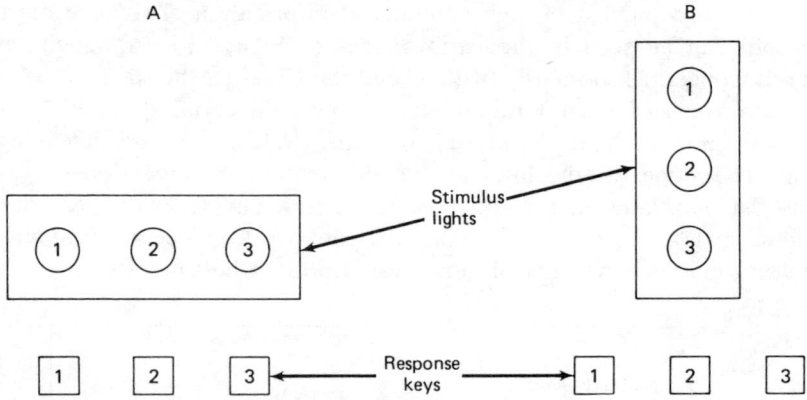

FIGURE 18   Two stimulus-response configurations differing in compatibility.

Stimulus-response compatibilty can simply be defined as the degree of correspondence between a signal or event and its correct response. The degree of correspondence can be defined as the extent to which the relationship between stimulus and response is seen by the majority of individuals to be the most natural or compatible. Consider the two stimulus-response relationships depicted in Figure 18. Configuration A demonstrates a natural one-to-one relationship between the stimuli, in this case lights, and the appropriate responses, which would be to press the key under the light that was presented. Configuration B, however, is not so straightforward, and involves some kind of mental manipulation to associate which light goes with which key. Although this is a relatively simple example of how compatibility can be varied, anyone wishing to construct the necessary components of these configurations can easily demonstrate that the reaction times to configuration B will be substantially greater than in the case of the more natural configuration.

Stimulus-response compatibility is precisely the variable that explains some of the differences between the slopes of the lines depicted in Figure 17. Tasks A through F represent stimulus-response relationships not too dissimilar from the example illustrated in Figure 16. Although there is a relatively well-defined relationship between each stimulus and each response, as the number of stimuli increase it becomes more difficult for subjects to keep the various stimulus-response relationships well defined, and hence their decision times tend to become longer. These results, when contrasted with the results of a classic study by Leonard (1959), however, readily demonstrate the importance of well-defined stimulus-response relationships. Leonard, in essence, demonstrated that if the relationship between stimulus and response is made very direct, the slope relating amount of information to reaction times becomes almost zero. His results (line J in Figure 17) were obtained by having subjects place their fingers on vibrators and, when they felt a vibration in one of their fingers, they were instructed to respond by pressing, with the appropriate finger, the vibrator that was vibrating. For two, four, and eight choices Leonard found that reaction time failed to get longer as it had in previous studies when event uncertainty was increased. Similar results were obtained by Mowbry (1960) when he studied a voice reaction to arabic numerals. These numerals were shown singly to the subjects and they responded by speaking the number concerned. Evidently, seeing a number and responding by saying it are highly compatible due to tremendous overlearning, and as a result the number of digits used (in this case groups of 2, 4, 6, 8, or all 10 digits were used) had no influence on reaction time, as is indicated by line G in Figure 17.

Another form of compatibility, which has important implications for the study of perceptual motor skills, deals with reactions to the spatial locations of stimuli. Simon (1969) found that his subjects had a tendency to react faster if the stimulus was located in the same direction as the subjects had to respond. This would indicate that an individual's expectations of where a signal will occur, and thus his preparation for a response in that direction, will have a facilitating effect on his reaction time. If he knows or can predict roughly where the signal will come from and can orientate and prepare himself to respond in that direction, his reaction time will be faster than if he were not prepared to react in that direction.

Another factor, related to stimulus-response compatibility, that considerably influences reaction time is the amount of practice an individual has on a given task, especially when there is poor compatibility. In one study, where the degree of compatibility was rather high, Mowbry and Rhoades (1959) studied how practice influenced responses that were made by keys under the subjects' fingers, with the corresponding signals for each key placed on a panel in the same pattern. Only two and four choice conditions were studied, but 42,000 trials of practice were given. After all this practice, performance in the four-choice condition improved to such an extent that it almost equaled that of the two-choice condition, even though initially the former condition was much slower than the latter. These results would seem to indicate that through practice individuals come to recognize more readily the correspondence between a number of responses and the individual signals that indicate that a specific response should be initiated and executed.

What are the implications of the above findings for perceptual-motor skills? In general, the stimulus-response compatibility research suggests that an individual must come to realize through instruction and practice what is required, in terms of action, when certain cues or signals appear either in the environment or through proprioceptive feedback. In essence, the performer must "map out" the association between these signals and the corresponding action. In certain cases, when there is high stimulus-response compatibility, relatively little instruction or practice will be necessary to bring reaction time to a minimum. However, usually for an individual learning an open skill, there are many potential events and cues that must be dealt with. With practice, the number of events that a performer actually deals with will decrease, since some events will be ruled out as not pertinent. Nevertheless, there will still be a considerable number of events and cues, each of which must be acted upon in a specific manner. Thus the performer must learn to match each of a considerable number of possible responses to specific situations that occur in the course of a game.

One interesting speculation regarding compatibility effects is that to develop compatible relationships a performer may be able to use mental practice. Whereas research has shown that mental practice is sometimes useful in improving performance of perceptual-motor skills, there is no evidence to indicate what causes the improvement. One possibility is that a performer, by viewing someone else perform a skill or by thinking about performing a skill, learns what responses are most appropriate for given situations. This would be a type of "game sense," and would be attributable to the development of stimulus-response compatibility. If research supports this speculation, teachers or coaches could facilitate the development of compatibility by directing their performers' attention to relevant relationships and instructing them, while resting on the sidelines or waiting their turn to play, to watch teammates in their position and attempt to anticipate what will happen. In this way, through mental practice, the performer not only must watch for relevant cues but also must anticipate the correct response. As a result, the decision process could be facilitated. The role that mental practice has in the performance and learning of perceptual-motor skills will be discussed further in Chapter 8.

Successively Presented Signals (The Psychological Refractory Period)

The last major factor that influences decision time to a signal or event concerns the situation in which two pertinent events occur in rapid succession. A practical situation where this occurs with a high degree of frequency is in games in which faking is an important part of skill execution. In basketball, for example, an offensive player often attempts to "lose" his opponent by faking in one direction and then immediately executing his intended movement in another direction. If the opponent has "taken" the fake, usually he is unable to recover fast enough to check the offensive player successfully. In psychological terms, the period involving the time it takes an individual to respond to a fake, realize that it is a fake when the real move of his opponent is recognized, and then initiate a response to the real move, is termed the psychological refractory period.

The psychological refractory period is illustrated in Figure 19 in a more systematic fashion. S_1 is the first signal and would represent the fake described above. If it is a good fake, it is assumed that the defensive player will react to it by selecting a plan of action and at least initiating movement to counteract the apparent move by the offensive performer. This reaction by the defensive player, which in essence is the time to perceive the signal, may ordinarily take from 200 to 400 milliseconds. This time interval is represented by the solid line between S_1 and R_1, where R_1 is the initiation of the response. During this reaction time period the offensive player initiates a second movement, S_2, and the defensive player must then process this signal while still reacting to S_1. As indicated by the time interval between S_2 and R_2, the time to react to the second event is considerably longer than the corresponding interval between S_1 and R_1.

Why is the reaction time to the second signal longer? It is thought that while a performer is processing a previous signal he is virtually in a state of refractoriness in that he is unable to process the information from a second signal simultaneously until the movement in response to the first signal is under way. This period of refractoriness is called the psychological refractory period, and is represented in Figure 19 by the dashed part of the line between S_2 and R_2. Thus it is this refractory period that is the cause of the considerably longer reaction time to the second signal.

A vast amount of research has been completed toward undertaking the psychological refractory period (for reviews see Smith, 1967; Fitts and

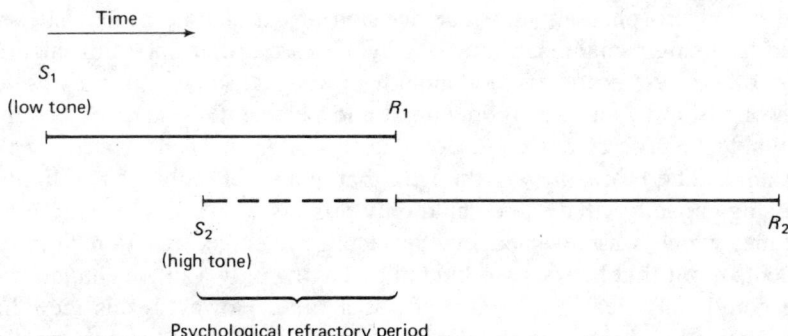

FIGURE 19 A schematic diagram of the psychological refractory period.

Posner, 1967; Welford, 1968; and Keele, 1973). This research has established the following facts about the psychological refractory period: (1) The reaction time to the first signal is almost always the same as when it occurs only by itself. (2) The reaction time to the second signal is almost always longer than when it is just presented as a single signal. (3) If the two signals are presented together, or at least within 100 milliseconds of each other, the performer may group them together and respond to them as a single signal, which sometimes eliminates the delay in response to the second stimulus. (4) Practice in itself does not eliminate the psychological refractory period (Gottsdanker and Stelmach, 1971). (5) The psychological refractory period can be eliminated if the performer knows in advance when and where the stimuli will occur and if he has considerable practice (Reynolds, 1966). (6) The psychological refractory period is not due to sensory or motor limitations, and therefore the delay is "central" in nature.

This last point is a very important consideration when attempting to determine the cause of the psychological refractory period. Research has indicated that the delay in response to the second signal is not due to a type of "physiological refractory period" corresponding to the inability of the nerve to recover from being fired, since this type of delay is known to be much shorter than the observed delays in the psychological refractory period. Similarly, it is not due to sensory or motor factors in that the delay occurs even when the two signals are presented through different sensory systems (for example, S_1 might be a light and S_2 might be a sound) and the responses are from two different systems (for example, R_1 might be a finger key lift and R_2 might be a voice response). Thus, the only remaining conclusion is that the psychological refractory period occurs somewhere in the central nervous system and most likely is a product of some attentional limitation.

In terms of trying to explain the central cause of the psychological refractory period, for many years the decision mechanism was thought to be the site of this phenomenon. The decision or translation mechanism was likened to a single channel, and it was hypothesized that once this channel was occupied by the processing demands of a signal (that is, searching for a plan of action to an already identified and pertinent signal), the channel was unable to process a second event until it was finished processing the first signal. Therefore, it was thought that man not only had a limited processing capacity (that is, he could only process so much information per unit time, which was revealed by the results of choice reaction time experiments), but that he was also limited by having only a single channel and hence could only deal with one event at a time. However, this view has been criticized as being too simplistic a view of the human performer. For one thing, in highly skilled performance, man certainly appears to be able to do several things simultaneously. For example, a highly skilled athlete not only can process cues from the environment and respond accordingly but he can also attend to the overall strategy of the game and be continually thinking about how to improve his and his teammate's position in regard to winning a point or a game. Thus it would appear that the concept of the single channel has its limitations in explaining highly complex behavior. To place the phenomenon of the psychological refractory period in its correct perspective in terms of the information processing activities of a human performer, a much more powerful concept of the decision process is required. This concept should not only be able to explain the psychological refractory period but also help to understand and explain the various factors, listed in this chapter, that influence decision times of the performer. Such a concept is now presented.

Time and Attention as Limiting Factors

At the beginning of this chapter it was pointed out that the responsibility of the decision mechanism was to select a plan of action in light of what the perceptual processes determine is the current state of affairs and what the objectives of the performer are. Selecting a plan of action is then seen as an attempt to reduce the discrepancy between what situations exist and what the performer wants. In terms of the information processing model, the major objective of this book is to determine what limits a performer's ability to process information. In the preceding chapter several perceptual limitations were noted, and in the present chapter it has been noted that several factors produce limitations in terms of time to process information. In general it was found that as the amount of information in the input was increased, the longer it took to decide eventually upon an appropriate response. In addition to the limitation of time, it was found that a second type of limitation existed in the form of the psychological refractory period. Here the limitation for making a decision was more of an interference type in that one signal interfered with or prevented the processing of a second signal presented shortly after the first one.

Keele (1973) recognizes these two types of limitations and postulates that they apply to all information processes in the performer. Limitations of time apply to all information processes, whether they be perceptual, decision, or movement in origin. The second type of limitation, noted above for the psychological refractory period, Keele ascribes to limitations of space. By space he means any information processing operation that requires part or all of the limited information processing capacity of the performer. If the reader remembers from Chapter 3, the performer has a limited amount of information processing capacity or attention, and if one task or mental operation requires part or all of this capacity, then the performance of a second task will be interfered with in the sense that there will not be enough capacity left to process the information from this second task. An important point concerning these two types of limitations is that some information processes may take considerable time but very little space. Consider a highly proficient basketball player dribbling a basketball. This act requires time but, since it is highly overlearned, requires very little attention, and thus the performer's attention can be used for processing other information demands from a basketball game.

To this point in the development of our information processing model (that is, the perceptual and decision mechanisms have been discussed) there have been instances where either or both time and attention limitations have applied to information processing activities in the perceptual and decision mechanisms. In many cases the amount of attention an information process demands is a function of practice. Take, for example, the identification of environmental events by the perceptual mechanism. As Keele (1973) points out, when there has been very little practice in a given situation, such an external event or signal will probably have a name attached to it, and after an event has been recognized, selection of a plan of action will proceed. In this instance, the perceptual process of recognition would take some of the performer's attention. However, after considerable practice it is conceivable that the name of a signal will not be a necessary mediator between the occurrence of that signal and selection of the correct plan of action. In this case, then, the perceptual process of recognition would take very little of the performer's information processing capacity.

Keele (1973) spends considerable time describing the limitations of information processing in the human performer. Instead of subdividing the information processes into perception, decision, and action, as has been done in this book, he considers only three processes: storage of information in memory; retrieval of information from memory; and the execution of movement in response to information. The information processes Keele includes under retrieval of information from memory are approximately analogous to the operations of the decision mechanism discussed in the present chapter. Keele's major point is that once enough information about specific situations in the environment and their appropriate responses to these situations is stored in memory, it appears that retrieval of that information demands very little, if any, of the performer's central processing capacity. Rather, it is the information processes that follow retrieval of information from memory that demand attention. These latter processes include initiation of movement, rehearsal, and some factors involved in movement control.

For our purposes it would appear that a combination of the three-component model (perception, decision, and action) with Keele's view would be most advantageous. Early in learning, when an individual is very naive about environmental events and appropriate responses, it may be that each processing stage is limited not only by time but also by attention demands. But once an individual's memory is well developed with the perceptual and response characteristics, as well as the various relationships between these two processes (stimulus-response compatibility), for any given skill or game the limitations of attention do not necessarily apply to all these processes.

The highly practiced individual, then, may be limited in performance in a way described by Keele (1973). Keele believes that event recognition, which sometimes requires time, requires no attention, and thus the performer can process more than one perceptual event at a time. Similarly, because the performer is highly practiced, perceptual identification and the selection of a plan of action are simultaneous. It is as if an event in the environment can be interpreted by the performer as requiring a given action without any intervening information processes. However, as Keele (1973) points out, a limitation occurs when a plan of action is initiated, as shown by work on the psychological refractory period, which never disappears with practice. This is taken as indicating that when a performer selects a plan of action, he must devote attention to this process, which will interfere with any other event also requiring attention. To this extent we can speak of the performer as being limited by a single information processing channel where the limitation is due to attention demands.

On the other hand, for the naive performer the translation of an input from the environment to an appropriate plan of action is not so smooth. Because of a lack of experience there are several information processing steps between input and output, each of which is limited by time and, in many cases, attention. Thus we might say that an inexperienced performer has several single information processing channels, each represented by the various stages that input information must be processed through. Again, it is appropriate to ascribe these limitations to a limited information capacity. At times the limitation might be perceptual in nature, when something in the environment might be difficult to recognize. Other times the limitation might be in the decision mechanism, where due to uncertainty the match of a signal to its appropriate plan of action takes both time and attention. Or the limitation could also be due to the initiation of a movement in a similar way to that described for the skilled performer.

In terms of the factors discussed in this chapter that limit an individual's decision ability it would appear that the limitations are due to both time and attention. Temporal and event uncertainty lead to limitations of time in performance in that the more uncertainty there is, the greater the time required for a response. It would appear also that for the naive performer there may also be a limitation due to the attention demands of this decision process. However, for the skilled performer this aspect of the decision process seems not to require attention even though it may require time, although even the limitation of time can be somewhat overcome by high amounts of practice or high stimulus-response compatibility. Thus the ultimate performance level, in terms of the ability to process information, would be achieved when a signal occurred in the environment followed by its immediate transformation into an appropriate plan of action, with a delay equal to about a simple reaction time.

Summary

This chapter has presented some of the processes that limit a performer's ability to make decisions. Reaction time was the variable that was equated with decision ability and it was shown that a performer has a definite limit to how much information he can process per unit of time. In this respect, however, it was seen that decision time was a direct function of amount of information in the environment rather than simply the number of signals or events. Moreover, though time to process information was seen as one factor that limited performance, the amount of attention demanded by a task was seen as another limitation. While all information processes require time, only some require attention, thus leading to a situation, in some cases, where a performer can process information from more than one source at the same time.

Suggested Readings

Measurement of Information

Attneave, F., *Applications of Information Theory to Psychology*. New York: Holt, Rinehart and Winston, 1959.

Fitts, P. M., and Posner, M. I., *Human Performance*. Belmont, Calif.: Brooks/Cole, 1967.

Keele, S. W., *Attention and Human Performance*. Pacific Palisades, Calif.: Goodyear, 1973.

Miller, G. A., The magical number seven plus or minus two: some limits on our capacity for processing information. *Psychological Review*, 1956, **63,** 81–97.

Information and Decision Times

Koster, W. G. (Ed.), *Attention and Performance II*. Amsterdam: North-Holland, 1969.

Welford, A. T., *Fundamentals of Skill*. London: Methuen, 1968.

Time and Attention as Limiting Factors

Kahneman, D., *Attention and Effort*. Englewood Cliffs, N.J.: Prentice-Hall, 1973.

Kerr, B., Processing demands during mental operations. *Memory and Cognition*, 1973, **1,** 401–412.

Posner, M. I. and Boies, S. J., Components of attention. *Psychological Review*, 1971, **78,** 391–408.

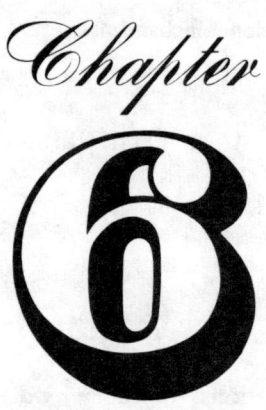

Chapter 6

The Effector Mechanism

The development of the information processing model presented in Figure 2 of Chapter 1 is now two-thirds complete. At this stage in the presentation of the model the information from the environment has been identified and classified, a perceptual response has been sent to the decision mechanism, and an appropriate plan of action has been selected. The effector mechanism can be seen as containing a large number of motor commands and, when a plan of action has been specified, must organize these commands so that the operations or movements they represent can be sent to the muscles in the correct sequential order. Thus a very large part of the operation of the effector mechanism concerns the effectiveness with which it can organize the various operations involved in a plan of action. Furthermore once it has organized these operations, its capacity for sending these commands to the muscles is also important in that some movements demand high amounts of information to be sent at a fast rate to the muscles in order that rapid movements can occur.

The purpose of this chapter will be to discuss two aspects of the effector mechanism. First, those factors that limit the rate of information processing (that is, the rate that commands can be organized and sent to the muscles) in the effector mechanism will be presented. Second, the way in which the motor commands are organized in light of a plan of action will be discussed.

Factors Limiting Information Processing in the Effector Mechanism

Amount of Information

The index of difficulty. In Chapter 5 considerable effort was made to describe how the amount of information affected reaction time. In general, as information in the input increased, due to increases in such things as temporal and event uncertainty, so did the reaction time. This was taken as indicating that the performer was limited by time in how much information he could process, and thus there appeared to be a definite capacity, for a given task at a given point in the learning process, for processing information. Paul Fitts (1954), rather than asking what the capacity of the decision process was, applied a similar analysis to a performer's effector mechanism. He reasoned that it was very difficult to study the motor system in isolation from the sensory aspects of performance but if "by asking [subject] to make rapid and uniform responses that have been highly overlearned, and by holding all relevant stimulus conditions constant with the exception of those resulting from [subject's] own movements, we can create an experimental situation in which it is reasonable to assume that performance is limited primarily by the capacity of the motor system." In such a situation, then, the only aspects of perceptual motor performance that would be stressed would be the operation of the effector mechanism and the visual and proprioceptive feedback loops that would permit a performer to monitor and control the movement.

To study the capacity of the motor system to process information Fitts constructed an apparatus similar to the one diagrammed in Figure 20. The subject's task was to take a stylus or pointer and, starting with the pointer on one of the targets, on a signal to start, move as rapidly and accurately as possible by alternately tapping each target until told to stop. By recording the number of taps and knowing the time subject was allowed to tap, a mean time for one movement from one target to the other could then be obtained. To vary the difficulty of the task, Fitts had several conditions where the width of the target was made smaller or larger and the amplitude of required movement made shorter or longer.

In the analysis of his results, Fitts used information theory to derive a formula that represented the difficulty of the task in bits of information. This binary index of difficulty, since called Fitts' law (Keele, 1968), is:

$$\text{Index of difficulty} = \log_2 \frac{2A}{W} \text{ bits/response}$$

By varying A and W, Fitts could thus increase or decrease the difficulty of a task and observe the effects of this on movement speed. His results showed

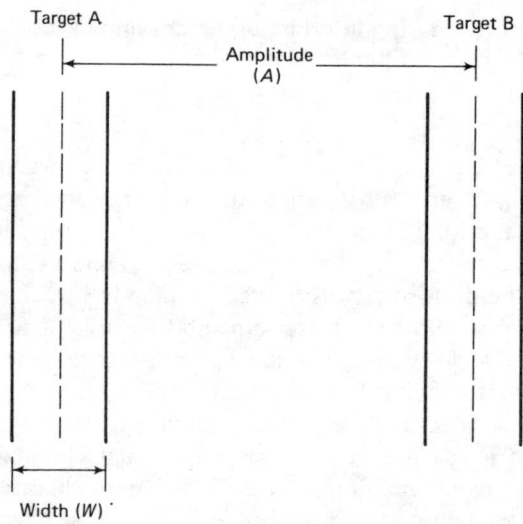

FIGURE 20 A version of Fitts' (1954) reciprocal tapping test.

a linear relationship between task difficulty and movement speed, with speed getting slower from an index of difficulty of one bit (180 milliseconds) to a difficulty of seven bits (731 milliseconds). These results were replicated in a later study (Fitts and Peterson, 1964) using a slightly different task, but the results again supported the fact that movement became slower with increases in task difficulty.

Although it is very difficult to generalize from Fitts' one-dimensional reciprocal tapping task to all types of movements, it is interesting to note that the above results show a definite capacity with which the motor system can process information. If there was no fixed capacity, movement speed should have been the same for each level of difficulty, but since movements became slower with increasing difficulty this indicated that a performer processes only so much information per unit time. The more information there is, the longer it takes to process it. The maximum rate with which the motor system can transmit information, as indicated in the above studies, was about 12 bits per second. Thus it would appear that just as the perceptual and decision mechanisms are limited by time to process information, the same limit of performance applies to the effector mechanism.

The effects of practice on the information processing capacity of the effector mechanism. The question of interest now concerns whether the capacity to process information reported above (about 12 bits per second), is a fixed value or whether it can be improved by practice. In Chapter 5, in which stimulus-response compatibility and practice effects were discussed in terms of how they influenced choice reaction time, it was found that these variables increased a performer's capacity to make decisions. In fact, if there was very high compatibility there appeared to be no limit in processing, since reaction time for relatively large amounts of information was just as fast as for low amounts of information.

Harry Kay (1962) conducted an experiment, the results of which bear on whether practice has an influence on the information processing capacity of the effector mechanism. His subjects' task was to pick up and place eight metal pins, each 1/8 inch in diameter, into metal holes. These holes varied in size from 9/64 inch to 72/64 inches, and the amplitude of movement to the hole varied from 2 inches to 16 inches. Thus, with these specifications, the index of difficulty for each of 16 specific versions of the task could be determined. Subjects then had 30 days of practice on each of the 16 tasks, performing each task once per day.

Over the 30 days of practice Kay found that there was considerable improvement in the information transmission rate of his subjects. Initially, his subjects performed at a rate of about 10 to 12 bits per second, which agreed with the earlier work of Fitts (1954), but some of his subjects achieved rates well over 20 bits per second in the later stages of the experiment. Kay concluded that this is a rather remarkable increase in just 30 days of practice, and predicted that for highly practiced subjects, like people who perform some industrial tasks of a similar nature for periods of years, the rate of information transmission would be considerably higher.

What is the cause of this tremendous improvement with practice? The answer probably can be found when one considers what effects practice has on the processing of feedback. To understand this fully, one must first consider what role the processing of feedback has in Fitts' law, and then considerations of what practice does to the processing of feedback during movement control will be more understandable.

Fitts' law and the processing of feedback in the control of movement. When a performer moves his body or a limb to a target or a specified position in space, one way in which he can be accurate is to monitor his movement continually by use of either visual or proprioceptive feedback, or both. In effect the performer compares the position of the body or limb, as it is moving, to the desired final location. If for some reason this comparison indicates that the current movement path is not correct, he can then modify it by executing a corrective movement. Thus by continually monitoring his performance through feedback, and issuing corrective movements based on this information, the performer can successfully move his body or limb to the desired location.

Although this description of movement seems plausible, it is too simple in that movements in most perceptual-motor skills are very rapid and the performer has only a small amount of time (in the order of milliseconds) in which to monitor his performance. The interesting question, then, is whether visual and proprioceptive feedback can be used in movements that are made rapidly and over relatively short distances.

The time to correct or modify movements has always been of interest to psychologists, perhaps because of their interest in trying to understand tracking skills, which form a large part of the total movement skills normally encountered by people. Driving a car, controlling an airplane, and many gunnery tasks can all be considered tracking in nature since rapid corrections of movement are necessary in order to perform the skill successfully. One obvious characteristic of tracking skills, however, is that the number of movement corrections is very limited. Early researchers, like Vince (1949), who studied the time it took to change directions of movements, found that approximately 500 milliseconds was required to process visual feedback. This would indicate that only two corrections per second could be made in the control of movement. This figure imposes a very severe limit, since many skilled movements are performed in much less time than 1 second. In essence this would mean that all movements less than 500 milliseconds in duration would be impossible to correct, and their final accuracy would be determined solely on the basis of the accuracy of the initial command to move.

A more recent study, however, has indicated that it takes much less than 500 milliseconds to make use of visual feedback in the control of an ongoing movement. Keele and Posner (1968) found this by studying a movement task that required subjects to move a stylus from one small circular target to another. The subjects were trained to move from one target to the other in 190, 260, 350, and 440 milliseconds. After they were consistently moving at these movement velocities, on some trials all the lights in the experimental room were turned off as soon as the movement was initiated. Thus the subjects, with the lights out, could not use vision in completing their movement. Keele and Posner then compared the accuracy of the movements made in the dark, at the various velocities reported above, to the appropriate movements made in the light. They found that the 190-millisecond movement was unaffected by being performed in the dark, whereas movements of 260 milliseconds were slightly more inaccurate, with the advantage of vision increasing as movement velocities became slower. Thus, the results indicated that subjects could not use visual feedback to control movements of 190 milliseconds, but for movements of 260 milliseconds or longer visual feedback was an effective means for reducing error. Keele and Posner concluded from these results that the time required to make movement corrections on the basis of visual feedback was between 190 and 260 milliseconds. This time is much shorter than that reported by

Vince, and indicates that vision may play a role in the control of relatively rapid movements.

As indicated earlier, another important source of information for controlling movement arises from proprioceptive feedback. A performer's "feel" of the path of his moving limb in a learned movement provides a stimulus upon which a correction can be based. A few experiments have attempted to determine the delay in response to a kinesthetic stimulus, and have found processing times faster than that required to process visual information. Chernikoff and Taylor (1952), for instance, found that it took only about 110 to 120 milliseconds for subjects to initiate a movement to reverse the direction of their arm when it was suddenly dropped from being passively held horizontally in a sling. Vince (1948) also provided evidence for the rapid processing of kinesthetic feedback. Her subjects were trained to pull a pointer down in response to a line that suddenly was displaced. On certain trials, unknown to the subjects, the tension of the pointer was increased and it thus took more effort to be pulled down. Vince found the time required to react to this increased tension was about 160 milliseconds.

From the above results it would appear that processing of kinesthetic feedback is faster than processing of visual feedback. A more important point, however, is that both types of feedback seem capable of being used to control movements of relatively short duration.

Even so, it should be apparent to the reader that movement control is not really continuous in nature in that corrections to movement can only be made once every 110 to 260 milliseconds, depending on whether the reaction is based on kinesthetic or visual information. This implies that for a good deal of the time that a limb or body is moving it is not under the direct conscious control of the central nervous system. Movement control, in essence, is a series of corrections, and between each pair of corrections the limb or body is not under conscious control. However, this does not mean that feedback is not being used during these periods. As will be seen later in this chapter, there is a very sophisticated feedback system, operating at the peripheral level (that is, between the muscles and spinal cord) and involving muscle spindles and muscles, that has considerable influence over the control of movement.

Returning to Fitts' law, and considering the above information on the speed with which feedback can be processed, it is now possible to postulate the processes that explain the relationship between the index of difficulty and movement time. This interpretation has been derived through the works of Crossman and Goodeve (1963) and Keele (1968, 1973), and involved postulating that the greater the task difficulty, the greater the number of corrections required to move accurately. To understand this, one must appreciate that according to Fitts' law a task can be made more difficult in either of two ways: by decreasing the target width or by increasing the amplitude of movement. As the difficulty of the task is increased in these ways, the performer must rely more on monitoring feedback, which leads to more movement corrections, and as a result the total movement time is increased. In fact, it is argued that if each movement correction takes approximately an equal amount of time, the total movement time to a target is simply the number of movement corrections multiplied by the time each correction takes.

From this interpretation, then, a movement to a target or location in space can be viewed as an initial movement and a series of movement corrections that eventually leads the body or limb to the desired position. Since processing of feedback takes time, the actual movement correction will not occur until after this processing time. Moreover, this interpretation of Fitts' law, while assuming that each movement correction takes an approximately equal time, also assumes that each correction leaves the performer with an error that is proportional to the distance remaining. This would imply that most of the movement time for a total movement is spent near the target. Annett, Golby, and Kay (1958) confirmed this prediction when they analyzed a film of performances on a task not too different from Fitts' reciprocal tapping task. They found that most of the movement time was spent in an area of about 2 inches in diameter about the target.

The final point to be made from the above analysis concerns the critical time in movement speed beyond which corrections, based on voluntary control, are impossible. It would seem that movements that last for less than about 200 milliseconds are unable to be controlled by visual feedback and, if they are less than 110 milliseconds in duration, even kinesthetic feedback cannot be used in their control.

Fitts' law, feedback, and practice. If Fitts' law describes the difficulty of a task in terms of the number of movement corrections required for an accurate movement, why is it that Kay (1962) found movement speed, for a given level of difficulty, to increase with practice? The implication would be that for well-practiced movements either the monitoring of feedback is not necessary or an individual monitors feedback but fewer movement corrections are necessary because of increased accuracy due to practice. It will be argued here that both explanations hold a certain degree of validity.

The argument is similar in concept to the one developed by Kay (1962, 1970) and essentially uses the idea that practice leads to redundancy in perceptual-motor skills. Consider a performer initially attempting a movement that is not familiar to him. Usually such a movement is performed relatively slowly and is characterized by a great deal of variability. Here the monitoring of the movement is done through both visual and kinesthetic feedback, which are compared to some external criteria for the movement. Through practice, the performer learns a great deal about these feedback signals until they eventually come to control his movement accurately. More importantly, however, because of this increased control, the feedback he is receiving from the movement becomes quite predictable in that the performer knows what a "good" movement should look and feel like. As a result of this, he is then able to predict in advance, perhaps even before he begins to move, what the feedback characteristics of the movement will be. If his movement is then executed as intended, the feedback from the movement, because it was expected, carries no information value in that it is redundant. This results in very little attention load to the limited information processing capacity of the individual. But if the feedback should deviate from the expected, the performer then has to bring his attention back to monitoring the feedback and thereby correcting his error.

In essence, because of this process the skilled performer has much less information to process in regard to control of a movement. He can probably set a critical bandwidth for allowable error in movement and, as long as the feedback remains within these limits, very little attention has to be spent on monitoring it. Now since a characteristic of highly skilled movement is that it is relatively accurate, this means not only that the skilled performer has a reduced information flow from feedback, but also that he will have fewer movement corrections to make in any given movement. Since the feedback interpretation of Fitts' law is based on the number of movement corrections it can be seen that the movement speed of a skilled performer will be faster because of fewer corrections. In conclusion, as was stated earlier, it would appear that practice not only allows a performer freedom from directly attending to the monitoring of feedback, but also leads to fewer movement corrections for any given movement.

Attention Demands of Movement Control

The monitoring of feedback, which leads to movement correction, as discussed above, obviously takes time, but it can be asked at this point just what evidence there is that indicates the attention demands of movement. In other words, the preceding section established the fact that movement control is limited by time and it also speculated that, except for highly skilled performers, movement control also seems to be limited by attention. The purpose of the present section, then, will be to explore just how movement control is limited by attention.

To say that movement is limited by attention is the same as saying that it requires all or a portion of the performer's limited information processing capacity. If this is the case, then it can be said, in terms already discussed in Chapters 3 and 5, that the movement requires space. It follows from this that if movement requires space, then a second attention-demanding task, performed simultaneously while a performer is moving, should be interfered with. This technique, used to determine whether movement requires space, is very similar to the psychological refractory period paradigm. Posner and Keele (1969) have called it the probe technique. It requires a subject to perform a primary movement task (for example, moving his preferred hand as quickly as possible to a target) and at the same time listen for a tone presented through earphones (the secondary or probe task) and react as quickly as possible, by pressing a button with his nonpreferred hand whenever the tone is presented. It is important in this technique that the subject attempt to perform the primary task as well as possible and attend to the tone only when it is presented. When this is the case, the degree to which the reaction time to the tone is impaired, compared to a control situation where the tone by itself is presented, can be taken as a measure of the attention demand of controlling the limb as it is traveling toward the target.

Figure 21 presents results from a probe study conducted by Posner and Keele (1969). They required their subjects to rotate a pointer on a knob (wrist rotation) to narrow or wide targets. The probe, a tone, was presented at random anywhere through the total range of movement. The mean control reaction time, represented by the straight line, was the time it

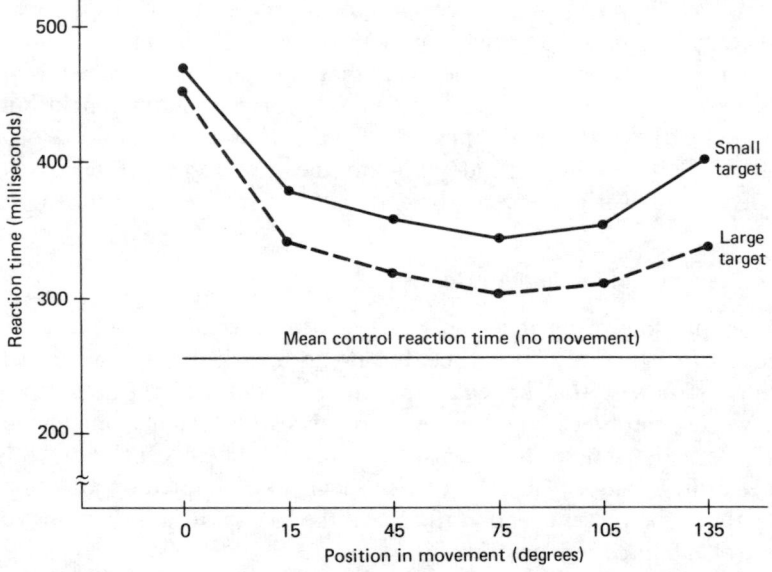

FIGURE 21 Attention demands of movement control (Posner and Keele, 1969. Reproduced by courtesy of Swets and Zeitlinger, from *Proceedings of the Sixteenth International Congress of Applied Psychology*, 1969, 419.).

took the subjects to react to the probe when they were not required to move the pointer simultaneously.

Posner and Keele's (1969) results, as depicted in Figure 22, revealed that probe reaction time was longer, for all movement positions, when subjects had to terminate their movement in the smaller target. Their results also indicated that the initiation and termination stages of movement required more attention in that a U-shaped function between probe position and reaction time was achieved for movements to both small and large targets. This finding may indicate that a subject is required to monitor feedback at the beginning and end of a movement more closely.

These results, especially the finding that movements near the target require greater attention demands, are consistent with the feedback interpretation of Fitts' law discussed previously. The finding that there was an attention demand early in the movement, however, is not consistent with this law since it predicts that there are very few movement corrections early in the movement. A possible explanation may be that the observed attention demand, rather than being due to the movement per se, was an indication of the processes involved in organizing and initiating the movement, and that the movement, once under way, required very little attention.

These results, however interesting, still do not yield any evidence as to the exact cause of the attention demand during movement. As Posner and Keele (1969) point out, there are two possibilities: First, the monitoring of feedback could take attention. Monitoring, in this sense, would be analogous to identifying the feedback perceptually and retrieving from memory an appropriate action that would correct any error signaled by the feedback. As Keele (1973) puts it, this is the memory retrieval stage of performance. The second cause of the attention demand could be due to the actual organization and initiation of the corrected movement or the response execution stage of performance.

To determine whether the attention demand of movement was caused by monitoring feedback or by the organization and initiation of a corrected movement, Posner and Keele (1969) contrasted two experimental movement conditions in which subjects were again required to react to the probe signal while performing the wrist rotation task described above. However, one condition involved blindfolded subjects who moved the pointer to a stop peg placed at the end of the movement. It was assumed that this type of movement would require processing of feedback, but would not involve any organization and initiation of movement corrections since the end point of the movement was specified by the stop peg. The other condition involved another group of blindfolded subjects, who moved the pointer to previously learned positions without the aid of the stop peg. Here, Posner and Keele reasoned that subjects not only would have to process feedback but also would have to use it for the purpose of organizing and initiating movement corrections.

The probe reaction time results of the above two conditions indicated that when subjects were required to move to the stop peg, the probe reaction times were the same as the control values. Posner and Keele concluded that monitoring of feedback, or the memory retrieval stage of performance, does not require attention. However, the second condition did produce slower probe reaction times. Thus it would appear that it is the movement initiation stage of performance that requires space.

These results on the attention limitations of movement corrections are almost identical to those results, discussed in Chapter 5, that indicated that for skilled performers the main attention limitation to performance was response initiation. In effect it was found that perceptual identification and response selection, what Keele (1973) refers to as memory retrieval, caused no attention demand. However, the same qualification that was discussed at that point is applicable to movement corrections; that is, for relatively unskilled performers the processes involved in perceiving feedback and then selecting a correction based on this perceptual process may take attention.

Control of "Continuous" Movement

As indicated in the above section on the limiting factors in the effector mechanism, control of movement is limited by both time and attention. It was established, for instance, that it takes at least 100 to 260 milliseconds either to initiate a movement or to correct a movement already in progress. The exact time required depends to a considerable extent on the type of stimulus, visual or kinesthetic, that the performer has to process. If these limitations are real, this should mean that the action of an individual who is required to make a series of movements, should be characterized by slow, jerky movements with relatively long time gaps between each movement. These time gaps would be caused by the necessity of the performer to process visual and kinesthetic feedback regarding his performance at each stage in the series of movements so that the next movement could be executed in terms of what happened in the previous movement.

The amazing thing about skilled performance, however, is that it is smooth and continuous in nature and it appears that the performer can make his movements with extreme flexibility and speed. In the previous section, it was seen that part of the reason for rapid movements was due to the redundancy of feedback achieved through much practice. This is, however, by no means the complete picture. Many perceptual-motor skills require complex movements, during which unexpected events can occur.

For example, a basketball player, ready to release the ball for a shot at the basket, can have his arm suddenly hit by an opposing player. Chances are that if the shooter is highly skilled, an immediate correction will occur and the shot will still be executed with considerable accuracy.

The purpose of this section of the book will be to describe the various factors that enable a highly skilled individual to overcome the limitations of information processing in terms of movement control so far noted in this book. Of particular interest will be how the performer overcomes the inherent delay in performance to reaction time and his ability to make very rapid movement corrections that are made too rapidly to be explained through voluntary or "conscious" control mechanisms. The topics that will be discussed in this regard concern the various levels of movement control that are known to exist within a performer's central nervous system, which range from highly voluntary to highly reflexive in nature, and how reaction time delays can be overcome through anticipation and the development of motor programs.

Levels of Movement Control

In the preceding section of this chapter the relatively slow reaction times to visual and kinesthetic feedback were discussed in terms of relatively discrete movements, like Fitts' reciprocal tapping task. Here, we are interested in studying complex series of movements that are performed very fast and where the use of visual and kinesthetic feedback, as previously described, is too slow to be used in its control.

However, the fact is that for an inexperienced performer this type of control is used. That is, the first of a series of movements may be initiated, the outcome analyzed through visual and kinesthetic feedback, and then the second movement in the series initiated, analyzed, and so forth, until the entire movement is completed. This type of movement control is called closed-loop control, where feedback is compared to some intended movement for the purpose of analyzing the correctness of the movement. If an error results, an attempt is made to correct the movement; if no error occurs, the next movement in the series of movements is initiated. This type of movement control, because it is both conscious and voluntary, is very limited in that, without anticipating feedback, the time required to evaluate the movement and initiate either a correction or another movement in a series of movements involves a reaction time. This type of movement control is characterized by relatively long delays between successive movements, and results in jerky, uncoordinated movement.

As well as having the above relatively long feedback loop to correct movement, there is another feedback loop that is known to operate considerably faster and without placing any attention demand on the central processing capacity. This is a reflexive feedback loop, consisting of feedback between the muscle spindles and muscles in the limbs. This lower-level motor control, termed alphagamma coactivation (Granit, 1972), allows a performer to adjust his movement in much less time than the larger feedback loop described earlier.

In Chapter 4, when kinesthesis was defined, some discussion was spent on describing muscle spindles, which are actually kinesthetic receptors embedded in the larger extrafusal or contracting muscles. Muscle spindles, however, are not strictly sensory receptors, for they can also be made to contract or relax by commands from the motor cortex via gamma motor neurons. The larger extrafusal fibers, of course, are controlled through alpha motor neurons. Thus, the motor cortex has direct control over both muscle spindles and extrafusal fibers.

It must be remembered, however, that the muscle spindles also have the qualities of sensory receptors in that when they are stretched they send nervous impulses to the spinal cord and brain via afferent neurons. The spindles can be stretched in two ways: first, since the two ends of each spindle are attached to the main muscle, if the main muscle is stretched without a corresponding relaxation of the spindle, the spindle would be stretched; second, the main muscle could be static or its shortening impeded if the limb to which it is attached is being impeded. In this case, if the spindle received the same motor command initially as the main muscle, it would continue to contract, and in the process would be stretched since its two ends are attached to the main muscle, which is either not shortening or shortening at a slower rate. In this manner, the muscle spindles serve as an error detector. As long as the spindle and the main muscle retain their relative lengths to one another no error signal is generated. But as soon as the discrepancy occurs between what is happening to the spindle and what is happening to the main muscle, the spindle discharges its error message into the spinal cord.

The last aspect of the interplay between the spindles and main muscles that must be described is the actual feedback loop that exists between them. When a spindle is stretched and sends its impulses to the spinal cord, these impulses are sent to the brain and, simultaneously, are fed back to the main muscles. The impulses going to the main muscles influence their contraction or relaxation in such a manner as to reduce the discrepancy between the length of the spindle and the main muscle. This latter feedback loop takes appreciably less time than the time required for feedback from the spindles to travel to the brain, be involved in a comparison from which an error results, and initiate a subsequent movement correction.

It can now be seen how closed-loop control of movement can take place at a relatively low level within the central nervous system. In essence, the original motor command to move is sent to both the main muscles and spindles. If muscular contraction occurs as indicated by the motor command, both the main muscle and spindles would contract together, thus maintaining a constant length between them and resulting in normal sensory discharge from the spindle. However, if the main muscle is perturbed in any way (unexpectedly stretched or relaxed) by the limb to which it is attached, a discrepancy between the spindles and main muscle will occur since the spindle will continue to assume the position indicated by the initial motor command. As a result, nervous impulses indicating this discrepancy will arise from the spindles, be fed back to the main muscle via the spinal cord, and operate on the main muscle to eliminate the discrepancy.

In this way, then, the muscle spindle actually represents the intended movement of the performer. By comparison of the intended movement with what is actually happening (the state of the main muscles), a continual closed-loop monitoring of performance can take place. This monitoring not only is a subconscious and automatic process, but also has the further advantage of being a relatively rapid way in which movement errors can be detected and corrected.

Two levels of movement control can now be appreciated. At the highest level are voluntary decisions based on comparing feedback to intended movement, which are limited by reaction times of about 100 to 260 milliseconds. To help fill in the time gap between successive reaction times is a lower level of control involving spinal level feedback control of movement. This lower level of control is quite rapid (of the order of 50 milliseconds) and presents no attention demands to the limited central processing capacity. Its main function is to correct small, unexpected discrepancies between intended movement and actual movement. In this way it is seen as a mechanism for smoothing out movement that occurs in the time interval between successive motor commands.

Although the above description of movement control helps us to understand how one motor command is executed in an efficient manner, it still does not answer the question of how a performer issues a series of commands in a short time interval that results in movements too fast to be controlled through a step-by-step analysis of visual or kinesthetic feedback.

Anticipation of Feedback

It is proposed that one way of eliminating the delays due to reaction time in the execution of a series of movements is through anticipation of feedback. This topic was discussed at some length in Chapter 4 and so will not be repeated here except to emphasize several points. The type of anticipation that a highly skilled performer probably uses in the execution of a series of movements is what was referred to as perceptual anticipation. Here, each component of a total movement must be initiated at the exact moment of completion of the previous component, and hence anticipation becomes an important aspect of performance. What the performer must do is anticipate the time it will take to complete the component he is currently executing so that he can begin to react to the second component in such a manner that the end of the reaction time coincides with the end of the movement of the previous component. In this way the movement of the next component would then begin without any time gap between the components.

Although this is a very viable mechanism for developing smooth, continuous movement control in that it eliminates the delay due to processing feedback, it still does not eliminate the attention demand of movement initiation. In other words, if a skill consisted of a sequence of movements, anticipating feedback from each movement would facilitate the initiation of the next movement in the sequence, but as was seen in the preceding section of this chapter, it would not eliminate the attention demand of initiating each movement. It stands to reason that a highly skilled performer cannot afford to attend to the initiation of movements because his attention is needed for such other things as analyzing the environment and attending to game strategy. Thus, the highly skilled performer's movement initiation and control must be highly automated and demand a minimum of attention. Since there is no question that this type of behavior is possible, as witnessed by the performance of a superior athlete, a different kind of control system must be operating. This more advanced control system can be envisaged as a motor program, and discussion now turns to this topic.

Motor Programs in the Execution of Movement

Rather than a performer continually having to monitor feedback for the purpose of controlling a movement, it has been proposed that through learning a performer has represented in memory an overlearned or fixed plan of action that specifies the sequential and temporal properties of a total skill. This fixed plan of action, when initiated, is capable of sending down a stream of motor commands that can control the entire movement independently of feedback. Thus the skill is said to be under motor program control, where the program refers to a fixed plan of action stored in memory. Moreover, every time this program is executed it is "run off" in exactly the same way, thus producing movements that have very little variability from time to time. This concept of the motor program is a rather speculative one in that there is only indirect research evidence for the existence of motor programs. There is no direct evidence that has shown that human performers can skillfully move in the absence of feedback or that they do not use feedback, even though it is present.

Perhaps the strongest support for the existence of motor programs comes from a study by Taub and Berman (1968), who surgically removed all proprioceptive feedback loops to the brain from the limbs of monkeys. After maximal recovery from the operation these animals were able to use their forelimbs for a number of tasks that required moderately rapid movements and that involved coordination with the hind limbs. This behavior also occurred despite the fact that a number of these monkeys were blindfolded, thus eliminating the possibility that they were relying on vision to control their movements.

Discussing the implications of these findings in terms of the central mechanisms that are responsible for such behavior, Taub and Berman (1968, p. 189) state:

Whatever the precise nature of the central mechanism responsible for the mediation of the phenomena observed in these experiments, we clearly have in them situations in which the CNS displays a considerable amount of autonomy and independence from the periphery in the acquisition and maintenance of behavior. Indeed, we could even say that the most general conclusion that can be drawn from our research is that in mammals, once a motor program has been written into the CNS, the specified behavior, having been initiated, can be performed without any reference to or guidance from the periphery.

In terms of human evidence, perhaps the strongest implication for motor programs in the performance of skills can be found in very rapid movements that last less than a reaction time (about 100 milliseconds), and which are made to stop at some target. This means that the movement is initiated, executed, and terminated at a target before feedback, either from vision or proprioception, can influence the movement, since the minimum time required for feedback to influence movement control is about 100 milliseconds. Thus, for the movement to be accurate this means that its initiation, execution, and termination must have been part of the motor commands sent down from the brain. These motor commands comprise what is known as a motor program in that it contains all the relevant information for motor control so that the sequence of commands can be carried out in the absence of feedback.

Although the above example serves to illustrate how a motor program operates over a very short interval of time, there is no reason why the motor program cannot be enlarged to include movements over a duration of 2 or 3 seconds. In this way, performance would tend to be relatively automatic and its attention demand would be quite small. It may be, however, that highly skilled performers use both motor programs and monitoring of feedback to control and correct their movements. These individuals may use motor programs to control most of their actions, but at the same time monitor feedback in a manner similar to that explained in a previous section of this chapter, entitled "Fitts' Law, Feedback and Practice." That is, because proprioceptive feedback is redundant for skilled performers, effective monitoring of this feedback takes very little of the limited information processing capacity. As suggested earlier, the performer might set a critical bandwidth for allowable error and as long as the feedback informs him that performance is within these tolerance limits, the performer can effectively execute his movements through motor program control. It is not until feedback informs him that relatively gross errors are being made that the performer must then consciously monitor and correct his movements. During this period, performance would probably be less well coordinated and slower. However, the skilled performer would soon bring his movements under motor program control, and performance would again return to a high degree of precision.

Hierarchical Organization and Control of Movement

The preceding sections of this chapter have discussed various ways in which movements can be controlled. We can now discuss these facts in a broader context, concerned with the basic principles of organization of the effector mechanism. The effector mechanism, as described previously, is basically involved in organizing and initiating a plan of action that was chosen by a performer in light of his goal and specific environmental conditions. The plan of action is analogous to what Miller, Galanter, and Pribram (1960) call a Plan, which they define as an organizational process that controls the order in which a sequence of operations is performed. Implied in this definition are the organizational principles of hierarchy and sequence and the fact that movements within a plan of action must be executed in relation to the plan.

Hierarchical and Sequential Organization

A plan of action can be considered a broad outline of the various operations that are necessary for a particular sequence of movements to be executed. The plan is hierarchically organized, which means that the various operations are categorized and then sequenced in terms of the order in which they are to be executed. An example of this process can be seen by considering the organization of the operations involved in the overhead clear in badminton, as shown in Figure 22. The plan of action for this skill would be an individual's idea of what the purpose of the clear is and what operations are involved in its execution, which presumably would initially be found by watching someone else perform the skill or by having a teacher explain and demonstrate it. The operations that are

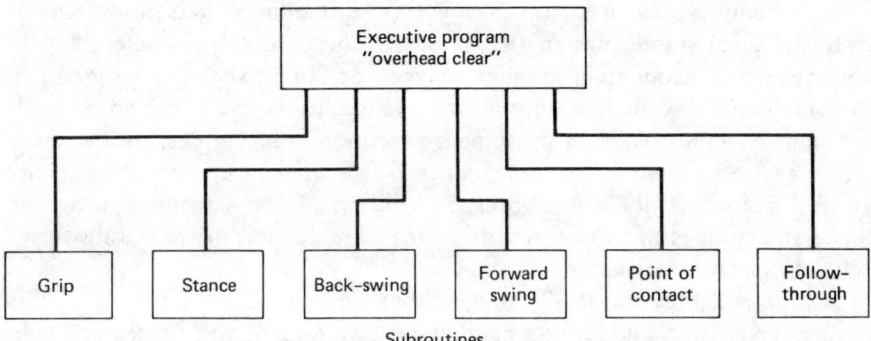

FIGURE 22 A computer analogy of the hierarchical and sequential organization of skill using as an example the overhead clear in badminton (Marteniuk, 1975b). From *Readings in Human Performance*, edited by H. T. A. Whiting (Lepus Books, London, 1975), with permission of the publishers.).

normally involved in the sequential execution of the clear are those concerned with the stance, grip, backswing, forward swing, point of contact and follow through. However, each of these operations is in essence a description of categories of smaller operations that must also have a sequential order if the larger operation is to be executed properly. For instance, the operations involved in executing the backswing would involve actions of the arm, shoulders, trunk, hips, and legs. Further, if one wished, each one of these latter operations could be seen as a sequential series of even more basic actions.

In this description of the overhead clear in badminton, then, a number of different levels of organization are apparent. At the top of organizational hierarchy is a broad plan of action. This plan can be broken down into relatively large operations that represent a less inclusive level of organization in that each one of these operations, in turn, is represented by another series of operations that are at still a lower level of organization. Presumably, one could describe even lower levels of operations that would be seen as basic operations involving such actions as grasping, pulling, pushing, and so on.

Thus, the badminton clear is seen as organized in a hierarchical fashion, with a definite sequence to which the operations, within this organizational framework, must be executed. In general, this type of organizational process is a characteristic of all skilled movement, and to develop further the implications this view has for studying perceptual-motor skills a computer analogy of the hierarchical and sequential organization of movement will be discussed. Fitts and Posner (1967) believe that the basic computer systems that are of importance in this analogy are the concepts of executive program and subroutines. The executive program is seen as being a plan of action that gives a particular skilled movement its overall logical framework in that it orders the execution of selected subroutines in a sequential manner. Moreover, the executive program is adaptable and flexible in nature in that changes to its structure can be made through detecting errors in movement execution. Subroutines, on the other hand, are seen as short, fixed sequences of movement commands that are run off automatically when ordered to do so by the executive program. Since subroutines are fixed in nature, they are capable of repeating themselves over and over again.

Fitts and Posner (1967) suggest that children past the first few years of life, given normal development, have acquired all the necessary subroutines to allow the learning of a wide variety of perceptual-motor skills. Thus, perceptual-motor learning, except in the very young, is seen as largely a matter of transferring subroutines from previously learned activities to a new executive program that gives an appropriate hierarchical and sequential order to these subroutines.

One important point about subroutines, which again emphasizes the hierarchical nature of skill, is that they may not have always been *fixed* sequences of motor commands. Initially, they may have been executive programs with a number of subroutines organized under them, and through learning the whole program has become fixed or automatic so that it is run off without conscious control. In this respect subroutines resemble the unconscious parts of movement, the control of which, because of learning, has been relegated to the lower centers of the brain.

In terms of our badminton example, then, the executive program is analogous to the idea or concept that a performer has about the specific operations involved in that skill. In helping a performer form an executive program, an instructor must make use of previously acquired movements (subroutines) so that they can be grouped under the new executive program. It stands to reason that in doing this an instructor must be aware of the past experience of his students. For instance, when teaching badminton, if the students have a wide variety of experience in other racket sports, their repertoire of subroutines that could be transferred to badminton will be considerably larger than students who have not had these experiences. In other words, because the experienced students have had an opportunity to learn appropriate movements involved in the basic components of racket sport (for example, stance, grip, action of the body while stroking), these movements have in essence become subroutines that can be transferred to a new activity. However, someone who has not had this experience will still have the necessary subroutines to perform the skill, but they will be at a simpler level of organization than those in experienced individuals. For example, while achieving and maintaining a correct stance during a given stroke in badminton can be considered a subroutine for an experienced player, for the inexperienced individual it is in essence an executive program containing a number of subroutines. Thus, this individual must work at a lower level of organization if he is to be successful in executing the stroke. In other words, while an instructor can give an inexperienced individual an executive program for a skill like the overhead clear in badminton, each of the major components of this skill might in essence be smaller executive programs that must be executed in a sequential manner. Each one of these smaller executive programs, while having fixed and automatic subroutines within them, would require considerable attention to be executed, thus adding considerably to the attention demand of the total skill.

This conceptualization of perceptual-motor skills in terms of executive programs and subroutines, which utilizes the principle of hierarchical organization, has a number of implications for teaching. Most important are the ways in which the past experience of learners is utilized in developing a new perceptual-motor skill and the way in which a teacher actually presents information about the new skill to an individual. More will be said about transfer of learning in Chapter 8 but at this point it will prove useful to consider the principle of hierarchical organization as it relates to how new material should be presented to individuals. Educational psychologists (Ausubel, 1967; Gagné, 1965; Lembo, 1969; and Rothkopf, 1965) believe that new learning material must first be broken down into essential concepts or principles and then ordered from simplest to most complex in a hierarchical fashion. Once this hierarchy is formed, the learner should be introduced to the new material at a level in the hierarchy appropriate to his past experience. The less past experience a learner has in the new material, the lower down the hierarchy he should begin in order that he will be dealing with material that is relatively specific and noninclusive. Once these lower levels of organization are mastered, however, the learner then attempts material at the next level in the hierarchy, and continues this process until the most complex and inclusive concepts are learned.

Ordering and introducing learning material in a hierarchical fashion has a number of advantages. First, it ensures that the learner can begin at a level most appropriate to his past experience and capabilities. Second, by attempting to organize material in a hierarchical fashion the instructor is forced to be systematic and logical in the organization and presentation of the material. This has a number of side benefits in that it increases the probability that correct prerequisites, to higher-order complex problems, are mastered by the learner before he attempts advanced subject matter. In addition, since the teacher is well organized and has the complete organizational framework of the material mastered, he is better able to provide appropriate sequences of inquiries and prompts for eliciting the correct behavior. Learning, from this viewpoint, thus becomes a developmental process and is more meaningful to the learner.

In terms of the above, it is proposed here that the computer analogy of perceptual-motor skills is an excellent way in which skills can be analyzed for the purpose of presenting them in an instructional situation. Not only will this force the teacher to become thoroughly familiar with the skill, but the question of where in the hierarchy instruction should begin is unavoidable. It also presents a logical framework to the student that will allow him to appreciate better the various operations involved in the correct execution of the skill.

Motor Programs and the Hierarchical Control of Movement

The preceding sections of this chapter have attempted to establish a concept of control of a series of movements based on the principles of hierarchical and sequential organization. It was seen that early in the development of movement control, feedback (visual and proprioceptive) was used as the chief means for detecting and correcting errors. However, through practice, motor programs were formed that specified all the parameters of the intended movement, and hence movement control was more of an automatic process. Nevertheless, even at this stage of performance, feedback was important in that it could be used to inform the performer of errors in movement. And it must not be forgotten that the closed-loop control of movement occurring between the main muscles and muscle spindles is a very important aspect of highly skilled performance.

This concept of motor control is directly compatible with the known hierarchical structure of the human nervous system. In essence, there are higher or conscious levels of the brain and lower or unconscious levels. Below the brain there is the spinal cord and the related reflex loops. Also characteristic of this organization is that different levels of the nervous system can acquire the capacity to act rather autonomously without the necessity of requiring attention. In the execution of perceptual-motor skills, then, the ultimate way in which a skill is performed would be to have it almost completely automated so that very little attention is required.

The research evidence showing the way in which perceptual-motor skills are brought under the control of unconscious control is rather meager, but one study does suggest that such a process occurs. Pew (1966) had his subjects attempt to keep a dot, which moved across a screen, centered on a line. This dot was continually in motion, and the subject could control its movement by pressing one of two keys with his index fingers. If he pressed one key, the dot accelerated to the left; if he pressed the other, the dot accelerated to the right. To keep the dot centered on the line the subject had to tap the keys alternately. Early in practice, the subjects used visual feedback to guide their performance in that they waited after a tap until they could see the dot accelerate in the appropriate direction. Then, upon seeing the error developing between the dot and the line, they would press the other key so that the dot would return back toward the line. Subjects made two or three taps per second at this stage in practice and their movements were quite jerky, with the result that there was only limited success. This type of control is characteristic of what was earlier called closed-loop control.

After several weeks of practice, however, there were signs that some subjects were developing motor programs. These subjects exhibited a very rapid and regular pattern of responding (of about 8 per second) and then, as the dot slowly moved away from the target a single correction would be made to bring it back on target, after which the rapid and regular pattern would be reinstated. This type of responding did not appear to be under visual control, but visual feedback was used periodically to effect a correction.

This experiment, then, demonstrates the theoretical process supposedly underlying the formation and execution of motor programs. Early in learning, performance is characterized by slow, jerky movements because of the necessity to use feedback for almost every response. However, once a motor program is formed, performance becomes rapid and coordinated, with feedback being used only periodically to correct relatively large errors in performance.

Pew's (1966) description of the formation of motor programs is also consistent with the computer analogy of perceptual-motor skills previously discussed in this chapter. The executive program, or plan of action, initially organizes the various operations that are necessary for the execution of the required movements. At the very lowest level of organization these operations involve highly overlearned subroutines, acquired from past experience, that represent motor commands that control very simple movements through the reflex loops of the spinal cord (that is, the muscle spindles and muscles). Depending on the extensiveness of an individual's past experience, these simple subroutines may or may not be subsumed under larger subroutines. If they are not, part of the learning process would be to group the very simple subroutines into several more inclusive "executive" programs. Through learning these executive programs would become overlearned and automatic and capable of being incorporated as subroutines, under some larger executive program. This learning process would continue until the executive program or plan of action for the entire skill was capable of controlling the entire hierarchical and sequential structure. This larger process would in essence be a motor program representing an overlearned plan of action. Every time this plan of action is selected by the decision mechanism, the various operations involved in it would be run off automatically and with very little attention demand.

Summary

The role of the effector mechanism in the performance of perceptual-motor skills was discussed. It was seen that movement control was limited by both time and attention. Time is a limiting factor in that the more information (as measured by the index of difficulty) a performer had to process about his movement, the slower the resulting movement. This limitation, it was argued, was due primarily to the inherent delay in processing visual and proprioceptive feedback for the purpose of controlling an ongoing movement. However, it was found that the capacity for transmitting information increased with practice. This increase in information processing ability was attributed to the performer's being able to predict in advance what the feedback characteristics of a movement are, thus making the actual feedback redundant and considerably reducing the attention demand of movement control. Furthermore, along with this decreased attention demand, practice was also seen as reducing the number of corrections required for the control of any given movement, thus resulting in an increase in the speed of the movement.

The second major factor limiting the information processing capacity of the effector mechanism, that of attention, limits movement control in that movement initiation demands attention, and as a result only one such operation can take place at a given time. In this respect it was shown that the actual monitoring of feedback appeared not to be attention-demanding.

Given the fact that movement control is limited by both time and attention, the next topic of discussion concerned how highly skilled performers seemed capable of overcoming these limitations in controlling their movements over extended time periods. To account for this, three types of movement control were discussed. First, a reflexive type of control involving the muscle spindles and muscles was seen as automatically and without any attention demand, smoothing out movements that were for some reason unexpectedly perturbed. Second, the prediction or anticipation of feedback from one segment of a movement was seen as a way for a performer to use this anticipated feedback to initiate the next segment of the movement. In this way the delay due to processing feedback was avoided, resulting in a sequence of movements with no time delays between them. Although this method of movement control is possible, it was pointed out that it still did not eliminate the limitation in movement initiation due to attention. Thus a third level of control, namely by motor programs, was discussed as one way a highly skilled performer could eliminate both time and attention limitations in the initiation and execution of a series of movements.

Although the discussion of movement as being limited by time and attention told a great deal about the capacity of a performer to control his movement, it told nothing about how movement information was organized within the effector mechanism. The latter part of the chapter was thus devoted to describing the hierarchical and sequential organization of motor skills and using a computer analogy to facilitate this description. Here, an executive program or a plan of action was thought to be a performer's overall idea of what was involved in a skill. Organized under this plan were subroutines, not too unlike motor programs, that represented fixed sequences of motor commands that could be run off automatically when called upon. This computer analogy of perceptual-motor skills was seen as being consistent not only with the way in which the human nervous system is designed, but also with the way in which motor skills are brought under the control of motor programs.

Suggested Readings

Factors Limiting Information Processing in the Effector Mechanism

Fitts, P. M., The information capacity of the human motor system in controlling the amplitude of movement. *Journal of Experimental Psychology,* 1954, **47,** 381–391.

Keele, S. W., and Posner, M. I., Processing of visual feedback in rapid movement. *Journal of Experimental Psychology,* 1968, **77,** 155–158.

Welford, A. T., *Fundamentals of Skill,* London: Methuen, 1968.

Control of "Continuous" Movement

Marteniuk, R. G., and Hayes, K., Kinesthetic information and the control of movement. In H. T. A. Whiting (Ed.), *Readings in Human Performance and Sports Psychology.* London: Lepus, 1975.

Posner, M. I., and Keele, S. W., Skill learning. In R. M. W. Travers (Ed.), *Handbook of Research on Teaching.* Washington, D.C.: American Educational Research Association, 1972.

Hierarchical Organization and Control of Movement

Gentile, A. M., A working model of skill acquisition with application to teaching. *Quest,* 1972, **17,** 3–23.

Lashley, K. S., The problem of serial order in behavior. In L. A. Jeffress

(Ed.), *Cerebral Mechanisms in Behavior: The Nixon Symposium.* New York: Wiley, 1951.

Miller, G. A., Galanter, E., and Pribram, K. H., *Plans and the Structure of Behavior.* New York: Holt, Rinehart and Winston, 1960.

Pew, R. W., Acquisition of hierarchical control over the temporal organization of a skill. *Journal of Experimental Psychology*, 1966, **71**, 764–771.

Pew, R. W., Human perceptual-motor performance. In B. H. Kantowitz (Ed.), *Human Information Processing: Tutorials in Performance and Cognition.* Hillsdale, N.J.: Erlbaum, 1974.

Section 3

Learning

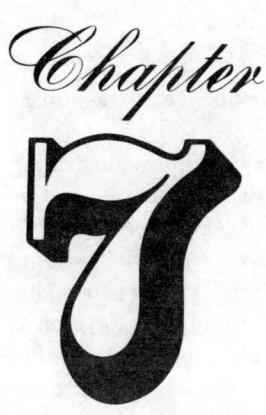

Information Processing in Perceptual-Motor Learning

Introduction

In Chapters 3, 4, 5, and 6 of this book the topic of learning was indirectly discussed through the concept of information theory. It was shown that perceptual-motor performance could be facilitated by reducing the amount of information that had to be processed by the central nervous system mechanisms. For instance, in the discussion of selective attention it was seen that a performer can effectively reduce the load of processing environmental information by learning to attend to only the relevant or pertinent cues. Further, expectations and redundancy also lead to a reduction in information processing in that if an environmental input is redundant it has no uncertainty attached to it, and thus it carries no information value.

While these processes were described for the perceptual mechanism it was also seen that similar processes were operating at the output or effector end of performance. In Chapter 6 it was noted that one of the main changes in performance occurring through practice was the ability of a performer to anticipate or predict the feedback from a movement about to be made. If the movement was executed as intended, the feedback was in essence redundant and as a result demanded very little of the limited information processing capacity. This process, however, was dependent on the ability of a performer to produce consistently a sequence of responses that matched the environmental demands.

An important common aspect of the above two examples illustrating facilitation of information processing, and of central concern to this chapter, is that both of these processes rely on memory. For perception to occur, incoming information must be compared to, or analyzed by, some process that is in the long-term memory store of the performer. This means that the performer, through experience and learning, has developed a perceptual memory that is capable of interpreting and recognizing incoming information.

Again, in a similar way, movement production is dependent on a memory system. The fact that a performer can organize and initiate a sequence of well-controlled movements, and retain these relatively well over long periods of time, implies that somewhere in his central nervous system is a permanent store of movement information. The way in which a performer develops this permanent store of information is called perceptual-motor learning.

The purpose of this chapter will be to study the processes involved in perceptual-motor learning. Unfortunately, space does not allow the treatment of perceptual learning since this is a complex and lengthy topic. If the reader is interested in this fascinating topic, he should read books by Haber (1969) and Lindsay and Norman (1972). Thus, in terms of the overall perspective of perceptual-motor skill learning, only one aspect of the three mechanisms will be covered in this book. That is, learning within the perceptual and decision mechanisms will not be discussed. The reader should keep in mind, however, that the processes of learning within these two mechanisms are very important in that they account for a large portion of performance in perceptual-motor activity. As Keele (1973) mentions, however, it may be that perception and decision can be understood as one process—that is, memory retrieval. Whatever the case may be, it is important not to lose sight of the fact that perceptual-motor learning is not just the learning of the output; rather, a complete description of learning would have to deal systematically with the underlying learning processes within each mechanism.

Conceptually then, the present chapter is more concerned with the output end of perceptual-motor behavior and more specifically with what information is used to form the permanent "motor" memory, and what factors influence a performer's ability to form this permanent store. In regard to these latter factors such topics as motor short-term memory, knowledge of results, knowledge of performance and motor programs are seen as important to the learning process and thus form an integral part of this chapter.

Performance Models That Incorporate the "Motor" Permanent Store

Before dealing with the specifics of motor memory, it will be of benefit to examine some of the recent models of perceptual-motor performance that have tried to account for the learning process. One such model was postulated by Laszlo and Bairstow (1971).

The standard in this model (Figure 23) is the total image or executive program of a given skill, and incorporates all the relevant information about the skill. As indicated, the learner acquires this information through instructions and situational cues, knowledge of results, and sensory feedback from kinesthesis, touch, vision, and audition as well as feedback from the motor command (efference copy). As Laszlo and Bairstow see it, this standard is not only important for storing information about the skill but is also important for controlling movement while actually executing the skill.

The motor programming unit, which is under the control of the standard, is analogous to a set of subroutines assembled for the purpose of executing the skill. The actual subroutines selected for the motor program are dependent on the amount of information contained in the standard. The more explicit the standard, the more suitable will be the selection of the subroutines.

The model, a closed-loop or servomechanism model of performance control, postulates that control of movement takes place by comparing sensory feedback and/or efference copy to the standard. This process

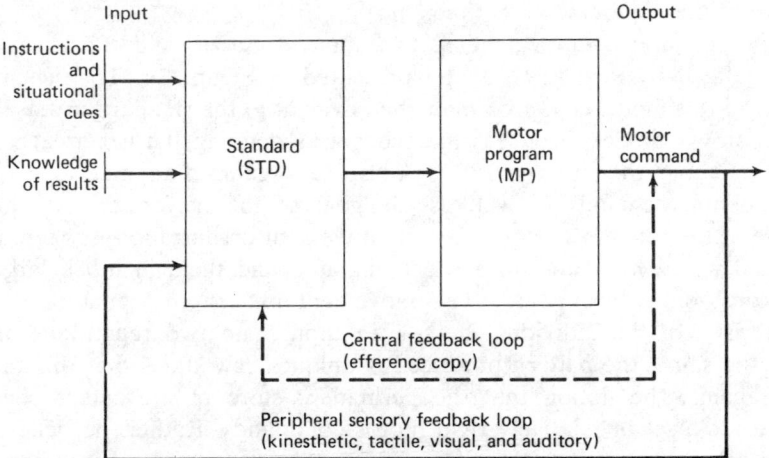

FIGURE 23 A model of motor learning and control (Laszlo and Bairstow, 1971).

allows comparison between the actual movement and the desired movement. If an error is detected, another movement is generated, which is designed to reduce the discrepancy of the initial one. Of course, this correction process is dependent on the limitations of time discussed in Chapter 6 and thus cannot explain control of very rapid movements (that is, movements lasting less than 200 milliseconds in duration). Movement in this latter case would be said to be under open-loop or preprogrammed control.

Laszlo and Bairstow incorporated efference copy into their model for two reasons. First, it provides an immediate comparison between the motor command (that is, what the movement will be like) and the intended movement through a central feedback loop. This feedback loop is much shorter than the peripheral sensory feedback loop, which means that a correction to a motor command could be initiated in a much shorter time than the times associated with the use of sensory feedback. Thus, error detection and correction could occur at a faster rate, which would enhance performance.

The second reason for the inclusion of efference copy in the model, and more important to the purpose of the present chapter, is to explain learning under conditions where no sensory feedback is available. In Chapter 6 a description was given of the work of Taub and Berman (1968), in which there deafferented monkey learned motor tasks in the complete absence of sensory feedback. To explain this, Laszlo and Bairstow postulate that the monkeys can use efferent information in a manner similar to the way in which sensory feedback is used in the development of the standard. It would appear, then, that a learner of a perceptual-motor skill has various sources of information by which to develop an image or standard of the requirements of that skill.

Another model, more detailed than that of Laszlo and Bairstow, is one postulated by Pew (1974) and presented in Figure 24. The schema memory of this model is approximately equivalent to the standard in Laszlo and Bairstow's model. Pew sees the schema as defining the general characteristics about the movement that must be organized to meet specific environmental demands as well as the goal of the performer. A good example of the role the schema plays in movement organization is when an individual writes his name on a sheet of paper and then, in much larger dimensions, on a blackboard. The movement pattern or signature is a characteristic of the individual and, even though no two repetitions are exactly the same, the pattern produced is unique. Pew states that this fact argues against the notion that the permanent store of movement characteristics is a set of relatively rigid motor commands. Rather, he believes that the schema represents properties of movement sequences, like spatial patterns, that are encoded and are applicable to a rather large range of specific movements with respect to a particular goal. In other words, using

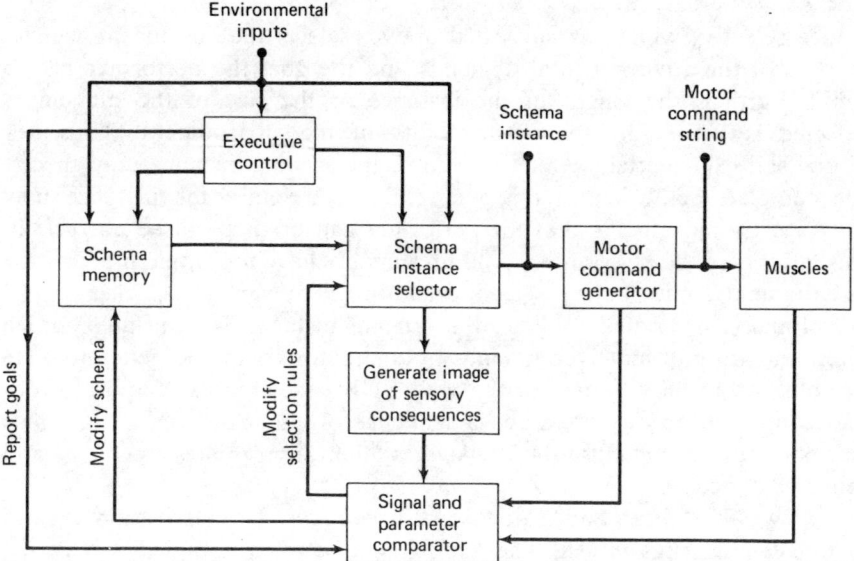

FIGURE 24 A model of motor learning and control that incorporates the concept of the schema (Pew, 1974).

the example of tennis, the tennis player has a schema for a forehand stroke, but the exact nature of the actual stroke for each specific time it is used is determined by the environmental conditions and where he wants to hit the ball. This explains, to a certain degree, why good tennis players probably never execute the same type of stroke in an identical manner from time to time in that the ball will never be in exactly the same position for each of these strokes. Thus the stroke must be modified to meet the exact requirements of the situation. Another example, illustrating the same point, is the quarterback in U.S. or Canadian football. To be an accurate and consistent passer, he must modify his passes to take into account the distance, velocity, and movement patterns of the receiver, wind and other weather conditions, and the particular defensive pattern with which he is faced. Obviously this requires subtle modifications of the movement pattern in the overarm throwing action used, and one might say a good quarterback would never throw the ball twice in exactly the same manner. The postulation of simple motor programs that control each throw thus becomes an academic exercise, since the quarterback would need a different one for each time he threw the ball. Rather, what is needed is a motor schema that, through experience and learning, comes to contain all the parameters that are needed to generate a unique movement to meet each situation.

The exact nature of the movement is determined by the schema instance selector, which, as suggested above, selects the specific movement in light of the environmental demands and the goal the performer has in mind. Further, the length of the instance or the size of the movement selected is limited by the predictability of the environment. Thus, for closed skills like certain gymnastic stunts, the schema instance may specify the complete act, whereas for open skills like tennis, the instance may only specify movements that the performer can predict will be correct. In this latter case the performer would presumably have to sample more of the environmental cues before selecting additional movements.

Finally, according to Pew, the schema instance is translated into a temporal string of motor commands by the motor command generator. He postulates that this segment of the model gives the skill its temporal order and can speed up or slow down a sequence of commands as a unit. This sequence of commands then activates the appropriate muscles, and movement occurs.

Pew, like Laszlo and Bairstow, also explains the closed-loop control of movement in his model. The comparison between intended and actual movements takes place in the signal and parameter comparator. This comparator receives information from various sources, which include: an image of the sensory consequences of the movement; information about the goal of the movement; proprioceptive information about the actual movement; and central information from the motor command. As in the Laszlo and Bairstow model, these sources of information are used both for movement control and learning processes.

Both of the above models, then, specify a number of sources of information that can be stored as a person acquires the ability to perform a skill. It would seem that he does not store specific motor programs that can be executed whenever needed; rather it seems that more abstract information about movement is gained through experience and the performer generates unique patterns of movement from this abstract store or schema to suit his specific needs. What is it that is actually stored in the schema? There is very little research available to base any discussion on, but the rest of this chapter will attempt to provide at least some direction to the answer.

Short-Term Motor Memory in Learning

According to the above models, the motor schema, which for our purposes can be called motor memory, receives information from various sources. Learning, or the establishment of a permanent motor schema, can be thought of as organizing this information into a meaningful structure. There are two important processes that determine the nature of this structure: one is short-term memory, in that all new information is subject to the limitations imposed by this system; the other process is the actual form of representation the information takes in the schema. This latter process is concerned with how a performer psychologically codes information, received from various sources discussed above, in memory. The way in which an individual codes information and the limitations of short-term memory, as discussed in previous chapters, determines the final representation of information in motor memory. It is to these two processes that discussion now turns.

In Chapter 5, in the section on time and attention as limiting factors, it was mentioned that Keele (1973) postulates three information processing activities that mediate input and output information: (1) storage of information in memory; (2) retrieval of information from memory; and (3) execution of a movement in response to information. Storage of information in memory, then, is the first step in the information processing chain of events. A learner must be capable of transforming information concerning performance into permanent representations that can be recalled at a later time. The form these representations take, as well as how time affects them, is of prime importance to the study of information processing in perceptual-motor learning.

Someone unable to code new information into some representation in memory presumably would never be able to use this information at a future time. In fact, Milner (1959) reports just such an example, in which an individual, having lost, through an operation for seizures, what appeared to be the area of the brain that housed short-term memory, failed to permanently retain any new information after the operation. Milner describes the subject as having difficulty finding his way home to a new house that he had moved into shortly before the operation. He was never able to remember where objects that are constantly in use, like the lawn mower, are kept even though he may have used it the previous day. In addition, he would read the same magazine over and over again without ever finding the contents familiar. Even though he had these difficulties with new information, his memory for events that were well learned before the operation was quite efficient. For instance, he had no trouble in remembering the address of his old house. How fortunate it is that the vast majority of people have a functioning short-term memory.

The present question of interest is to examine how an individual processes movement information so that it can be retained for short intervals and, in the process of this short-term retention, eventually transforms the information into a more permanent form. In other words, we are interested in the learning process. Before describing coding processes in motor short-term memory, it will be beneficial to examine the processes found for certain types of nonmotor information. This short diversion

162   Learning

will provide a conceptual framework by which motor memory can be studied.

Figure 25 presents a schematic representation of one way in which visual information has been found to be processed from the time it is received by an individual's visual receptors until it is finally represented in long-term memory. The first form or representation for visual information, depicted in Figure 25, is short-term sensory storage, which is a very short-lasting direct representation of the presented material, with a persistence of approximately 1 to 2 seconds (Mackworth, 1963). To be retained past a time interval of 1 or 2 seconds, the visual information in this sensory store must be recoded or transformed into another form that represents short-term memory. This second representation is still relatively unstable in that it can only be retained in this form for approximately 20 to 30 seconds. Keele (1973) summarizes evidence to show that one form of representation that visual information takes in short-term memory is auditory in nature. One way this was determined was by observing that recall errors of subjects, approximately 30 seconds after they were presented with visual material, were characterized by auditory confusions. In other words, it seems that visual information is recoded into an auditory form and stored in short-term memory, where forgetting can occur because of interference or confusion among similar-sounding representations.

If the information in short-term memory is to be retained for longer than 20 to 30 seconds it must be recoded again into a more permanent form called long-term memory (see Figure 25). Keele (1973) again shows that one form that information in long-term memory takes, despite the fact that it was initially visual in nature, is a semantic form. It seems that individuals store the meaning of the information in long-term memory, and thus errors of recall are primarily related to the meaning of the original material.

Although the above description of the passage of information from short-term sensory storage, through short-term memory to long-term mem-

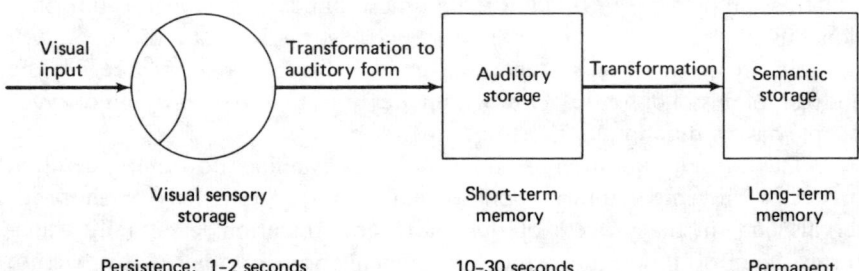

FIGURE 25   Information processing stages involved in storing visual information in memory (Marteniuk, 1975. From *Readings in Human Performance*, edited by H. T. A. Whiting (Lepus Books, London, 1975), with permission of the publishers.).

ory, represents one possible way in which information is represented in the various stages of memory, there are many other possible alternative forms. As Keele (1973) points out, there appear to be a large number of individual differences in the way information is coded and recoded in the three types of memory systems. However, if we are ever to understand the memory process, the strategies of how people code input information must be further studied. And it is exactly this type of analysis that must be done in relation to how individuals code movement-related information.

Unfortunately, the state of knowledge on how movement-related information is coded in memory is nowhere near the corresponding state of knowledge concerning visual and auditory information. However, there are some studies that are suggestive as to the nature of the motor short-term memory code, and it is to this topic that we now turn. In addition, in a later section of this chapter, the topic of the motor schema or permanent motor memory will be discussed.

In reviewing the work of Adams and Dijkstra (1966) and Bilodeau, Sulzer, and Levy (1962), as well as interpreting the results of his own study, Posner (1967) postulated that an image may be the form that movement-related information takes in short-term motor memory. Posner (1967) defined an image as a relatively direct nonverbal representation of the input information, which could possibly be in the form of a spatial map containing all relevant information about the movement. The strongest evidence for this viewpoint comes from Posner's (1967) own results from his examination of retention of movement information that had been presented to subjects either while they were blindfolded or while they could see their movements. The subjects attempted to reproduce movement distances ranging in amplitudes of up to 90 degrees. The standard movement was presented to them by having them move a lever to a stop, and then, after an appropriate retention interval, they were required to reproduce the movement but this time without the aid of the stop. In addition, during the reproduction movement the subjects were required to reproduce either the end location of the standard or the distance (amplitude) of the standard. For this latter condition Posner (1967), by a random method, made the starting position of the reproduction movement different from the starting position of the standard movement, and the subjects had to reproduce the amplitude of the standard movement. Thus they could not use the location cues of the standard movement as a guide in their reproduction movements.

Posner's results showed that when subjects were blindfolded their reproduction movements became worse over the 20-second retention interval (see Figure 26). This was so even though some subjects were allowed to sit quietly during the retention interval (that is, the rest condition). It was also true whether they were required to classify digit pairs into high

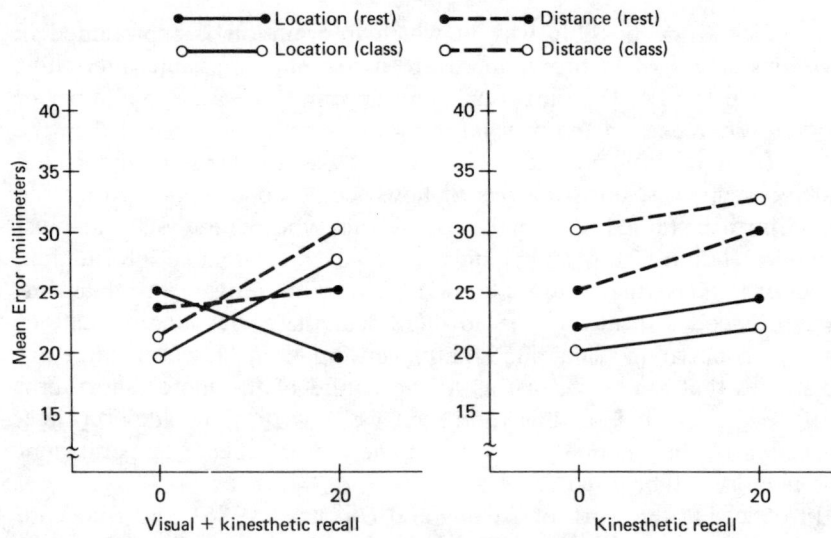

FIGURE 26 Short-term memory retention characteristics of visual and kinesthetic information and kinesthetic information (Posner, 1967. Copyright 1967 by the American Psychological Association. Reprinted by permission.).

or low and odd or even (the classify condition). However, when subjects were allowed to see their movements, different results were obtained in that those subjects that were required to reproduce the end location of the standard movement did not forget over the retention interval that involved resting for 20 seconds.

Posner interpreted this latter finding as evidence for movement information being stored in the form of an image. Not only were the subjects extremely accurate in their reproductions, but many of them reported using imagery as a guide in retention and reproduction. Furthermore, it seems that location information would be better suited for imagery because it would be capable of being placed in a spatial map to a greater extent than would distance or amplitude information.

The fact that Posner's (1967) blindfolded subjects all demonstrated forgetting even over an unfilled retention interval is surprising, but it does perhaps indicate that kinesthetic information, in order to be retained, must be first combined with information from another sensory system. In essence, information from vision might be used to "calibrate" or organize the kinesthetic information, thus allowing it to be retained over an unfilled retention interval. Without the aid of vision, however, kinesthetic information would be unable to be retained and would be spontaneously forgotten.

Another study that lends support to the notion that location information is perhaps remembered because of a subject's ability to place it into a spatial map (that is, the image) is one by Laabs (1973). He contrasted the ability of blindfolded subjects to retain either location or distance information over a 12-second retention interval.

His results (Figure 27) indicated that subjects who rested over the 12-second retention interval were able to retain the location information, but forgot or did worse when they were required to retain distance information. Thus it would appear from this study that subjects can somehow use location information in the form of an image so that this information can be retained over an unfilled retention interval. One word of caution, however, is appropriate before accepting the results of the studies by Posner (1967) and Laabs (1973) with any great certainty. In reporting their results, Posner used, as his index of forgetting, absolute error (the mean of the errors without taking into account their algebraic sign) while Laabs used, as his index, variable error (the standard deviation of the algebraic error of a subject's repeated efforts to reproduce a standard movement). This obviously limits the conclusions that can be derived from these two studies, since performance was measured differently in each case. The reader should be aware of differences in these two types of errors and is referred to a paper by Schutz and Roy (1973) for this information.

Besides the difficulties of interpreting differences in the two types of error measurements in the above studies, another complicating issue becomes apparent from the results of a study by Marteniuk (1973). He again studied the differences in retention between location and distance information, but this time, as indicated by Figure 28, found that both types of information could be retained over an unfilled retention interval. This would indicate that under certain circumstances distance information is also able to be represented in a form that is capable of being stored and retained in short-term motor memory. How this form differs from the idea of an image and its relationship to location cues will have to await further investigation.

While the image has been postulated to be at least one important way

Delay	Reproduction cue	
	Location	Distance
Immediate	3.64	3.93
Rest (12 seconds)	3.72	5.01

FIGURE 27 Short-term memory retention characteristics of kinesthetic location and distance cues (Laabs, 1973. Copyright 1973 by the American Psychological Association. Reprinted by permission.).

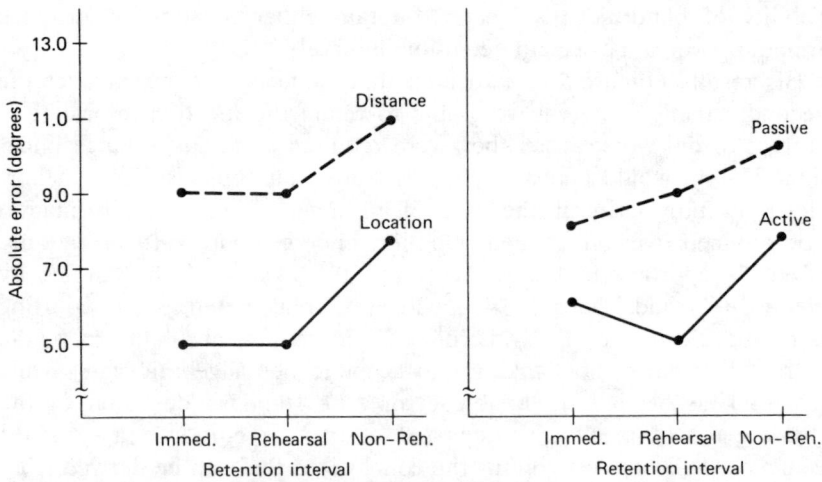

FIGURE 28 Short-term memory retention characteristics of several kinesthetic cues over three retention intervals (Marteniuk, 1973).

of retaining movement information in short-term memory, another factor that is related to this notion is the concept of organization and its influence on memory. As Keele (1973) has discussed, not only is the form in which information is represented in memory important, but also the way in which these representations are organized is crucial to the retention process. For instance, in the retention of verbal items it has been found that while imagery is one method used to retain the verbal items, those people that are able to structure or organize these images in some specific way demonstrate superior retention compared to those individuals that have no method of structuring their images.

Although there is no work in motor short-term memory that demonstrates how the organization of images influences movement retention, there are two studies that show how organization of movement information presented to subjects affects their recall of this information. The first study, by Nacson, Jaeger, and Gentile (1972), used as its theoretical base the premise that an individual actively engages in attempting to organize incoming information. In essence, they rejected the traditional notion that a subject just passively receives information from his external environment and internally produced sensations. Rather, the subject will attempt to utilize his past experiences in actively manipulating this input information into an organizational framework that is easily retained and recalled. Nacson et al (1972) found support for this idea when they discovered that the ability of subjects to reproduce arm positions without the aid of vision was enhanced when they were given special verbal instructions about the nature of the movements prior to the movements being presented. The instructions were concerned with describing where the end positions of the movements to be reproduced were and how these positions related to each other.

The idea that organization can affect the retention of movement was further supported in a second study by Nacson (1973). This time no special instructions were given to the subjects, but instead the order of presentation of the five standard movements was varied among several groups of subjects. The order of presentation varied from the case in which one group was presented the five standards in a completely random order to the case in which a group was presented with the smallest movement first, then the next largest, and so on until all five movements were presented and recalled. There were two other groups in Nacson's study, in which the variability in the order of presentation of the standard movements was somewhere between the two groups previously described. In essence, Nacson was manipulating the organization of input information by varying the order of presentation of the standards: the highest level of organization was represented by the systematic presentation of the standards from smallest to largest, with the least amount of input information organization occurring in the group of subjects who were presented the standards in a random order.

Nacson's (1973) results confirm the notion that organization of input information affects retention of movement information in that the best recall performance occurred for the group that had been presented the standards in a systematic fashion, whereas the poorest performance was associated with the random presentation of standards. However, although these results are certainly very meaningful in that they show the importance of input information organization on recall of movement information, there are other considerations that future work in this area will have to concern itself with. One concern deals with whether Nacson's (1973) study on organization really manipulated organization of memory codes. For instance, one rival interpretation might be that the group presented with standards in a systematic fashion actually had less information (that is, less uncertainty) to process and therefore it was easier to retain and recall this information. The group that was presented the standards in a random order, on the other hand, had the maximum amount of uncertainty or information to process and therefore, from an information processing viewpoint, their task was the most difficult. Another issue related to this concerns the difference between experimenter-produced organization and subject-produced organization. Both of the above studies (Nacson et al., 1972; Nacson, 1973) varied organization through experimenter instructions or the method by which the experimenter presented the standard movements. If the way in which subjects code information is of central concern, the interest should be in discovering the way in which subjects naturally attempt to code and organize movement information. As was pointed out earlier in this section, the verbal and visual literature shows that there appears to be considerable individual differences in the way subjects represent these kinds of information in memory. The same will probably hold for movement information, and thus different methods of investigation (that is, other than manipulating experimenter-produced organization) will have to be devised to study these individual differences.

The Schema as Motor Memory

The two preceding sections of this chapter introduced, respectively, the concept of the schema and properties of motor short-term memory in terms of coding information. The purpose of this section is to propose that the schema can actually be thought of as motor memory having short-term characteristics, as described in Chapter 4.

As early as 1932 Bartlett (1961) was describing the concept of the schema as the basis for a theory of remembering. His description and definition of schema was:

. . . an active organization of past reactions, or of past experience, which must always be supposed to be operating in any well-adapted organic response. That is, whenever there is any order or regularity of behavior, a particular response is possible only because it is related to other responses which have been serially organized, yet which operate, not simply as individual members coming one after another, but as a unitary mass. Determination by schemata is the most fundamental of all the ways in which we can be influenced by reactions and experiences which occurred some time in the past. All incoming impulses of a certain kind, or mode, go together to build up an active, organized setting: visual, auditory, various types of cutaneous impulses and the like, at a relatively low level; all the experiences connected by a common interest: in sport, in literature, history, art, science, philosophy, and so on, on a higher level. There is not the slightest reason, however, to suppose that each set of incoming impulses, each new group of experiences persists as an isolated member of some passive patchwork. They have to be regarded as constituents of living, momentary settings belonging to the organisms, or to whatever parts of the organism are concerned in making a response of a given kind, and not as a number of individual events somehow strung together and stored within the organism.

Suppose I am making a stroke in a quick game, such as tennis or cricket. How I make the stroke depends on the relating of certain new experiences, most of them visual, to other immediately preceding visual experiences and to my posture, or balance of posture, at the moment. . . . When I make the stroke I do not, as a matter of fact, produce something absolutely new, and

I never merely repeat something old. The stroke is literally manufactured out of the living visual and postural "schemata" of the movement and their interrelations. I may say, I may think that I reproduce exactly a series of textbook movements, but demonstrably I do not; just as, under other circumstances, I may say and think that I reproduce exactly some isolated event which I want to remember, and again demonstrably I do not.

Continuing on from this last sentence, Bartlett makes the point that memory must not be thought of as a reduplicative or reproductive event. Rather, memory should be thought of as constructive in nature where, as in the tennis example, each stroke is built up on the basis of the immediately preceding balance of postures and the demands of the game. Thus from this viewpoint, Bartlett's concept of producing a unique motor act is similar to Pew's (1974) treatment of schema and "schema instance." The "schema instance" is the end result of the constructive process that results when an individual has to act in some specific way. In particular, then, these concepts can be used to explain a large range of open skills where execution is dependent on the environment. These concepts also suggest that the idea of motor programs, as discussed in Chapter 6, are much too simple to account for the flexibility of motor behavior. It is obvious that skilled individuals could not achieve the tremendous number of different movements required in a complex game just through the use of a finite store of fixed motor patterns or motor programs. To appreciate this, one just has to watch a tennis player, who receives balls from a wide range of different angles, trajectories, and speeds, and whose bodily postures are always in a different position as he begins to make a stroke, and yet who can place the ball within the relatively small area of his opponent's court with, at times, a high degree of accuracy.

The Development of the Schema

How does an individual acquire the rich store of experience necessary for a schema that is flexible enough to generate an almost limitless number of instances adapted to specific environmental demands? Hebb (1949) believes that this type of behavior, which he calls motor equivalance, depends on the simultaneous occurrence during learning of perceptual information about the goal of the motor behavior (for example, seeing a ball coming toward you and realizing when and where you have to hit it) and the particular sensory consequences of the motor activity that an individual employs to achieve the goal. Hebb postulates that, through learning, the perceptual information about a skill becomes internalized so that a skilled individual "intellectualizes" the skill and uses this thinking process, in conjunction with feedback from his movement, to control the achievement of any specific environmental demand. Thus the "intellectualized" part of the skill or, in other words, the schema, is the highest level of control and, through feedback and the various lower control loops discussed in Chapter 6 and this chapter, an individual has a great deal of flexibility in adapting his movement.

Lashley (1951) has attempted to account for the motor equivalence problem by postulating "space coordinate systems" that controlled movement. This type of control system, again similar if not identical to Bartlett's and Hebb's viewpoints, depends on internalized spatial representation of the axes of the body and of gravity as well as the space coordinate systems of the environment derived primarily through vision, audition, and touch. In essence, the integrated knowledge of the body and environment, gained through experience, are stored in a spatial coordinate system and can be used to specify the exact movement necessary to accomplish a specific goal.

The motor schema, then, is seen as incorporating all the above ideas with the main purpose of explaining the high degree of flexibility of skilled motor behavior. While Hebb talks about the internalization of perceptual experiences and Lashley postulates an internalized spatial coordinate system, the exact makeup of the schema is still unknown. Research has not yet established the exact properties of a movement sequence that are encoded and become intrinsic to a particular schema. One line of research that is making some progress in this direction, however, is that dealing with the characteristics of intersensory integration.

Intersensory Integration and the Schema

The schema, as outlined above, is some form of internalized representation of an individual's past experience that allows him to generate unique sequences of motor commands. Bartlett, Hebb, and Lashley, as presented above, all speak of the schema as an organized store of integrated sensory information. This implies that the schema is not entirely "motor" in nature but rather relies on an integration of information from all the sensory systems. Birch and Lefford (1967) and Connolly (1969), while agreeing with this concept, believe that the integration between the visual and kinesthetic systems plays the major role in the development of voluntary motor control.

Intersensory integration is usually manifested in what has been termed cross-modal equivalence. This is an individual's ability to judge accurately the equivalence or nonequivalence of sensory input to two or more different sensory modalities. For instance, an example of proprioceptive-visual cross-modal matching would be for an individual to feel the length of a rod placed in his hands, and then attempt to identify that rod visually when it is placed, with three or four others of varying length, before him. If he is accurate in picking out the correct rod over a number of trials he would be considered to have established an equivalence between the proprioceptive and visual sensory systems. The fact that this equivalence is present implies that somewhere in the brain there is an integration between the visual and proprioceptive sensory areas.

It is proposed here that the schema responsible for producing flexible and adaptive motor behavior is based on a rich store of highly organized and integrated information developed through experience and through the simultaneous occurrence of information in the various sensory systems concerned with perceptual-motor performance. This concept, developed behaviorally by such researchers as Bartlett, Hebb, and Lashley, has been recognized as being neurophysiologically sound in that it has been shown that one of the primary functions of the central nervous system is the integration of sensory information. In essence the central nervous system integrates sensory information received simultaneously from the various sensory systems by establishing associative networks within the associative area of the sensory cortex (Konorski, 1967).

Intersensory integration seems to play a very large role in the development of information processing abilities in children. Birch and Lefford (1967), in studying cross-modal equivalence of visual and tactile-kinesthetic information of children, found that the capacity for integrating this kind of information improved during the ages of six to eight. Along with the development of this sensory integration ability these authors also noted a parallel increase in the child's ability to regulate his overt motor behavior. They found that at ages five and six about 40 percent of the ability to perform a perceptual-motor skill (reproducing geometric forms) was accounted for by a child's intersensory integration capacities, whereas at ages seven and eight about 55 percent of the perceptual-motor skill was explained by intersensory integration ability. These authors concluded that improvements in intersensory integration and in perceptual-motor skill are due to an increased liaison between the senses.

Although studies of intersensory integration in children are supportive of the idea that a schema underlies the development of perceptual-motor skills, they do not tell us very much about the specific way in which sensory information is integrated to produce skilled movements. To understand the mechanisms of motor learning more detailed knowledge is needed about the relationship between visual and proprioceptive processing.

Connolly and Jones (1970) and Jones and Connolly (1970) provide just such knowledge in that they systematically studied visual and kinesthetic sensory integration in children and adults. Their experimental task involved having the subjects reproduce lines of varying length, which they could do in four different ways. In the first condition, vision to vision (V-V), the subjects viewed the length of line to be reproduced (the standard), and when it was taken away the experimenter presented a line to the subject by slowly extending a metal tape. When the subject thought the tape was the same length as the standard line he told the experimenter to stop, at which point an error between the standard line and the reproduced line was noted by the experimenter. Thus in this condition the subject only had visual information to base his judgments upon. The second condition, kinesthesis to kinesthesis (K-K), required the *blindfolded* subject to produce the standard by moving a pointer along a smooth slot in the apparatus until the pointer was opposed by a stop placed on the slot. This represented the standard length and it was based only on kinesthetic information. The subject was then required, while still blindfolded, to return to the starting position and then move along the slot to a point where he thought the end location of the standard length was. For this reproduction the stop was removed. Again an error between the standard length and the reproduced length was recorded. Obviously, this reproduction was based entirely on kinesthetic information.

The third and fourth conditions were designed to study the cross-modal equivalence of vision and kinesthesis. In the third condition, vision to kinesthesis (V-K), the subject was presented the standard line visually, as in condition one, but was required to reproduce it kinesthetically, that is, as in condition two where he was blindfolded and had to move the pointer along the slot. Here, the subject had to match a visual standard with kinesthetic feedback he received while moving his arm to reproduce the standard. If vision and kinesthesis were integrated, one would expect that this cross-modal equivalence task would produce relatively small errors. The fourth and final condition of this study was just the opposite of the third one. Here the subject was presented the standard kinesthetically as in condition two and for reproduction purposes was required to make a visual judgment as to when the tape, extended by the experimenter, matched the standard length, as in condition one. Again, this condition (K-V) measured cross-modal equivalence between vision and kinesthesis, but this time in the reverse manner as in condition three.

Conditions three and four, then, were designed to measure the degree to which intersensory integration had been developed in the subjects. The first two conditions were intramodal comparisons, and past research indicated that these types of comparisons were usually more accurate than cross-modal comparisons. Presumably this is so because comparisons within a sense are simpler and do not require the transfer of information, a more difficult process, between sensory systems. The results of this study proved this latter point to be valid in that the intramodal performances were superior to the cross-modal performances. In addition it was found that the V-V condition was superior to the K-K condition. In terms of reproduction ability and age, this experiment confirmed earlier work in that performance, for both intra- and cross-modal comparisons, increased with age. The age groups studied were groups whose mean ages were approximately 5 years, 8 years, 11 years, and 23 years.

The most interesting result of Connolly and Jones' study, in terms of the purpose of this chapter, was a marked discrepancy between the V-K and K-V conditions. It was shown that there was an asymmetry in cross-modal comparisons in that the K-V condition resulted in less error than the V-K performance. It appeared that kinesthetic information was capable of being translated into visual information whereas subjects were unable to perform as well when the reverse process was required—that is, when visual information had to be translated into kinesthetic information.

To account for this asymmetry Connolly and Jones proposed a model of perceptual-motor learning presented in Figure 29. They assume the visual and kinesthetic information each have their separate short-term memory systems and that translation between these modalities is dependent upon the integrated long-term store, or in our terms, the schema. They postulate, and offer as evidence the study of Posner (1967) (presented in the immediately preceding section of this chapter), that visual short-term storage is more efficient than the kinesthetic store. Posner found that when an individual was given the opportunity to rehearse visual information it could be readily retained, whereas this was not true for kinesthetic information.

Posner's findings serve as a basis for Connolly and Jones' most significant proposal in the model they present. They predict that in a task

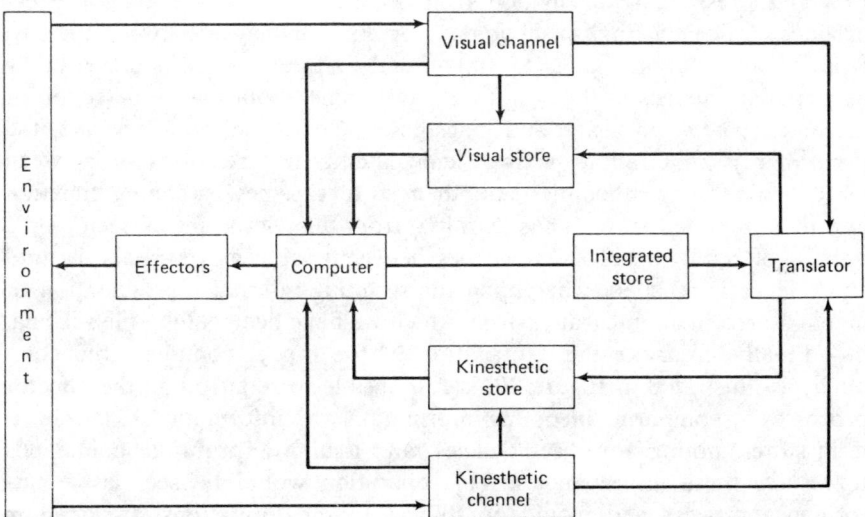

FIGURE 29 A short-term memory model based on intersensory integration of visual and kinesthetic information (Connolly and Jones, 1970).

requiring cross-model matching the translation of information between modalities takes place prior to its being put into short-term memory. This means that for a task dependent on intersensory integration, like V-K, the visual input is translated into a kinesthetic code and it is stored in kinesthetic short-term memory until it is used in producing a response. Similarly, in a K-V task, the kinesthetic signal is translated into a visual code and stored in visual short-term memory. Of course in intramodal tasks, kinesthetic and visual inputs are stored as such in their appropriate memory stores.

According to Connolly and Jones, the reason the V-K condition is not as accurate as the K-V condition is the inherent instability of the kinesthetic short-term memory store. As Posner found, and his results were confirmed by Jones and Connolly (1970), information stored in this memory system is subject to spontaneous forgetting even when the central processing capacity is unoccupied.

Other important features of Connolly and Jones' model concerns their concept of the long-term integrated store. They believe that it contains some internal representation of the relationship between visual and kinesthetic information. These internal representations are initially formed by visual and kinesthetic inputs occurring simultaneously (for example, watching and feeling your hand move to a target), being equated or collated, and then passed on to the long-term store. Connolly and Jones, in explaining the collating process, use the analogy of English and French dictionaries, where English might represent information from vision with French representing information from kinesthesis. The collating process produces a French-English dictionary, or an equivalance between the two types of information that is the integrated long-term store. Further, they believe that changes in the long-term store come about by the detection of mismatches between vision and kinesthesis. When a mismatch occurs, the performer is required to actively calculate a new relationship between these two sensory modalities and then store this new mapping function into the integrated store. Thus learning, from this viewpoint, is seen as the process of reduction of discrepancies between vision and kinesthesis until equivalence is reached, whereupon the resulting internal representation or map is stored in an integrated store, which we have been calling the schema.

Finally, to make the explanation of the model complete, the computer, as illustrated in Figure 29, is responsible for controlling the effector processes by comparing incoming information with information in the short-term stores, noting any discrepancies, and issuing appropriate commands to resolve these discrepancies. This operation would be seen as a performance process and would be subject to the limitations discussed in Chapter 6.

The major implication that can be derived from the above discussion in terms of the mechanisms underlying perceptual-motor learning concerns the role of vision in learning. It has long been known that vision is the dominant sense, and it appears from the above discussion that vision acts to quantify or organize kinesthetic input. One can think of vision as being the process that calibrates kinesthetic information so that it can be stored in a meaningful manner and recalled for future use. One would predict from this that kinesthetic information that is unable to be coded in this fashion would be subject to spontaneous forgetting and thus would be useful for only very short periods of time after it was received. This may explain some of the discrepancies among the studies reported in the discussion of motor short-term memory in this chapter. For instance, the work on the short-term memory for kinesthetic location cues shows that this information can be retained over an unfilled interval, whereas distance information is not retained as well or at all. It may be that location cues are more easily coded into a visual representation and thus retained to a greater degree. In this respect, location cues may form the basis of the spatial coordinate system postulated by Lashley (1951) to underlie the control of movement. In fact, this contention was supported in a study by Attneave and Benson (1969), who found that vision was the necessary prerequisite to the accurate coding of tactual information into spatial information. Thus it appears that there is a substantial amount of work to support the contention that the development of the motor schema, while relying somewhat on proprioceptive information (for example, aspects of kinesthesis, touch), is dependent primarily on visual information. It is dependent on visual information to the extent that vision provides a means of mapping or coding proprioceptive information into the internal representational system called the motor schema.

One other important issue raised in the above discussion concerns the postulation of the integrated store or schema as one of the basic mechanisms underlying perceptual-motor learning. Research to date has shown that the integration of vision and kinesthesis appears to be very necessary for perceptual-motor learning, but the question remains whether other types of sensory information are not equally important for the schema. For instance, major league baseball catchers have often been reported as saying that they can determine the exact nature of a hit by the sound the ball makes when it contacts the bat. Expert squash players sometimes get confused when they are prevented from hearing the sounds a squash ball makes when it hits the opponent's racket or when it hits the wall. Obviously, much more research is needed to determine the exact nature of the schema.

The Concept of the Motor Program Redefined

In Chapter 6 the idea of motor programs was discussed and defined. In general it was thought that, through learning, performers acquire fixed sequences of movements, called motor programs, that when called upon execute movements in an identical manner time and time again. Motor programs were postulated to be present in skilled performance primarily because of the rather speculative evidence indicating that performance can occur in the complete absence of feedback.

Proponents of motor programming theory postulate that an individual acquires a motor program for every specific act that he encounters in the execution of skilled movement. Since this seems plausible for closed skills, since usually these skills must be performed in an identical manner each time, the motor programming theory fails when it has to account for open-skill behavior. In open skills, since no two situations (for example, two underhand forehand strokes in tennis) are ever exactly the same because of a variable environment and an endless number of positions of the performer's body and limbs prior to the stroke, motor programming theory would have to predict a separate motor program for each one of these movements. Not only is this unreasonable from the point of view that an infinite number of programs would be required, but the learner would never be able to acquire the program in the first place since no situation ever repeats itself. This latter point, of course, assumes that repetition of performance is necessary before a motor program can be formed. Surely, then, the concept of motor programs as highly overlearned sequences of action, stored somewhere in the brain for future use, must be viewed with extreme skepticism.

The concept put forward here is that the control of skilled perceptual-motor activity starts at a very high level in the central nervous system with the motor schema, and control proceeds through a series of control loops, each one of which becomes more direct and simple in function. In essence, perceptual-motor behavior is viewed as a hierarchy of levels of organization, as described by Miller, Galanter, and Pribram (1960), which in effect implies a hierarchy of control loops as discussed in Chapter 6.

An important assumption of this view of motor control is that feedback is a necessary part of the process. However, the extent to which feedback is used is primarily a function of the type of skill and the level of learning. Performance of closed skills can perhaps have a minimum of feedback involved since, through learning, a performer can generate a relatively long sequence of movements without monitoring feedback because of the static nature of the environment.

Although open skills, because of their varying environment, always demand a match between the exact environmental demands and movement, this still does not mean that feedback has to be utilized constantly. As reviewed in Chapter 6, the study by Pew (1966) indicated that performers are capable of producing relatively long sequences of movement without directly referring to feedback. Undoubtedly, anticipation of environmental signals as well as movements, which lessens the information load, also plays a crucial role in the control of complex skills.

Although we could take specific aspects of the total control system (for example, the schema instance) and call it a motor program (implying that performance occurs in the absence of feedback), we would probably be correct if we observed performance only over a short time interval. This was pointed out in Chapter 6, where it was stated that a movement that is started and stopped in an interval of less than 100 milliseconds must be under the control of a motor program since there is insufficient time to use feedback in its control. However, this is surely not the type of perceptual-motor behavior one observes in real-life situations. Most skills are of much longer duration than this and are much more complex in nature. Thus, to understand the control processes involved in such behavior one must look for a flexible and adaptive system and appreciate the many processes involved. When one combines the notion of the motor schema, as established in this chapter, with many of the information processing principles discussed in the previous chapters, one is closer to realizing some of the factors involved in highly skilled performance.

Knowledge of Results and Performance

The Role of Knowledge of Results and Knowledge of Performance in Learning

Up until now, most of this book in discussing feedback has primarily explained the processes and limitations involved in how an individual uses feedback to control and evaluate his performance. Evaluation, almost exclusively, has been taken to mean the comparison of feedback (for example, proprioception and vision) to the intended movement. As defined in Chapter 1, this type of feedback is called knowledge of performance.

When studying purposeful movement (that is, goal-oriented movement) another dimension of feedback must be discussed. This second dimension of feedback is called knowledge of results, and entails a comparison between what a movement accomplished (that is, the outcome) and what the original goal was. For example, a basketball player who executes a shot can see the result of his action (where the ball goes) and can compare this result with the original goal (sink the ball in the basket). Knowledge of results is important to learning in that, as indicated by both the Pew and the Laszlo and Bairstow models presented earlier in this chapter, this is at least one way in which the schema is modified. Of interest also is the fact that knowledge of results, like knowledge of performance, can be augmented. In other words, the learner can not only receive these two types of feedback through his own sensory system, but this feedback can also be augmented by a teacher or coach informing the learner about the execution of the movement (augmented knowledge of performance) or by interpreting the process of movement in attaining the goal (augmented knowledge of results).

		(Knowledge of performance) Was the movement executed as planned?	
		Yes	No
(Knowledge or results) Was the goal accomplished?	Yes	Get the idea of the movement	Surprise
	No	Something's wrong	Everything's wrong

FIGURE 30 The use of knowledge of performance and results in evaluating motor performance (Gentile, 1972).

Obviously both knowledge of performance and knowledge of results are important to the learning process. Gentile (1972), in her model of skill acquisition, clearly points out the need for these two types of feedback in the evaluative process underlying the learning of perceptual-motor skills. Figure 30 presents the four rather simplified decisions that Gentile sees a performer making after each attempt at the performance of a skill. If the relatively naive learner, after executing a skill, decides that both the movement was executed as planned and the goal was accomplished, presumably he would proceed to become more sophisticated in terms of the degree of accuracy required both for his movement and its result. If the goal is not attained but the learner felt he made the correct movement there is probably something wrong with his idea about the movement required to accomplish the goal. In essence, he has generated an inappropriate schema instance or sequence of motor commands, and although he intended to make the correct movement, he was not successful in attaining the goal. Through augmented knowledge of results from the teacher or coach, the learner may be given insight into what type of movement is correct.

If the learner feels that he executed the movement incorrectly but still accomplishes the goal (he receives a surprise answer) any one of a number of things could happen. For one, he could modify his movement plan or schema instance in an attempt to bring the executed movement into line with the planned or ideal movement. Another alternative would be that the learner continues to repeat the incorrect movement pattern, since it did accomplish the goal, but in this situation he runs a risk of developing a skill that is probably rather limited in the ultimate degree of success. An example of this situation would be an inefficient jump shot in basketball (for example, not jumping very high or perhaps releasing the ball from a point outside of the shoulder instead of from the midline of the body). What the learner must recognize, if this is the case, is that this performance, though initially successful, will ultimately limit his performance at later stages of learning. Therefore the teacher must work at attempting to bring the initial plan for movement and movement execution into congruence. Here, augmented knowledge of performance would be an essential type of feedback for the teacher to give the learner in order that this change will occur.

As Gentile points out the last possible result of the evaluative process, the No/No cell in Figure 30, could lead to a number of different decisions, which could include the decision to quit—especially if this result were achieved in several successive attempts. In this case the learner can systematically attempt to revise his motor command, perhaps change his goal or attempt to reevaluate completely the relationship between the goal and required movement. However, in the end he may be at the mercy of the teacher or coach in that augmented knowledge of performance and results may be necessary for the learner to make any progress at all.

Principles of Use of Knowledge of Results and Performance

Since the foregoing section indicates that knowledge of results and performance seem to be rather important for the learning of perceptual-motor skills, it will be beneficial to review some of the research literature that deals with this topic. In particular, it will be of interest to determine how essential it really is for learning, how precise it has to be to influence learning, the frequency with which augmented feedback should be given to maximize learning, and when in the learning of a movement it should be given. However, two points on the following discussion should be appreciated. First, this discussion deals with knowledge of results in a way that is different from what a teacher or coach would encounter in a practical situation. Most of the studies to be reviewed use experimental motor learning tasks in which a subject cannot normally receive knowledge of results by himself. For example, a favorite experimental task used in the study of knowledge of results has been a positioning task, where a blindfolded subject is required to reproduce some standard movement length. Since he is blindfolded, he is unable to compare the outcome of his reproduction movement with the standard movement length he was attempting to reproduce. In this situation the experimenter usually verbally tells the subject how well he did, and this is called knowledge of results. In a practical situation, such as shooting a basketball, the learner usually has his own knowledge of results (that is, he can see the outcome of his attempt) and he could also receive augmented knowledge of results from the teacher. The point is, then, that the reader should keep this distinction clear when reading the following review. Practically, there may be times (especially in the early learning phase) when a learner is unable to accurately determine the outcome of his movement, and augmented knowledge of results will be necessary. In this case the reader will see that the principles for the use of the feedback are quite clear. However, when a learner has both his own knowledge of results present as well as augmented knowledge of results, the straight application of these principles lacks experimental verification and, until the proper experiments are conducted, the practitioner should consider the use of these principles as only guidelines.

The second point that the reader should keep in mind while reading this review on knowledge of results, is that the same principles probably apply to the use of augmented knowledge of performance but, again, there is no research literature to indicate that this is so. Therefore while the general principles discussed are informative and useful, when a teacher or coach wants to know how to use augmented feedback, it must be stressed that these principles are only guidelines and that their actual verification awaits further research, especially in light of the two points discussed here.

Thus, with these qualifications established, the following principles for the use of augmented feedback in perceptual-motor learning can now be presented.

Knowledge of results is necessary for learning. A well-established fact is that if a learner is not told how well or poorly his movement matched the goal or desired outcome, learning will not occur. A study by Trowbridge and Cason (1932) demonstrated that if subjects are not able to assess their errors in performance, no learning occurs. These authors studied the ability of blindfolded subjects to draw a 3-inch line and found that the performance of a group of subjects who were not told anything about their errors failed to improve or get worse over 100 trials of practice (see Figure 31). The results of this group were in marked contrast to two other groups of subjects, who received different types of knowledge of results (KR). One of these groups was given *qualitative* knowledge of results (they were simply told by the experimenter whether their movement was right or wrong) while the other group was given *quantitative* knowledge of results (the subjects were told their errors by the experimenter giving numbers that corresponded to the number of 1/8-inch units in the error). For example, if the experimenter said "plus 2," this represented an overshoot of

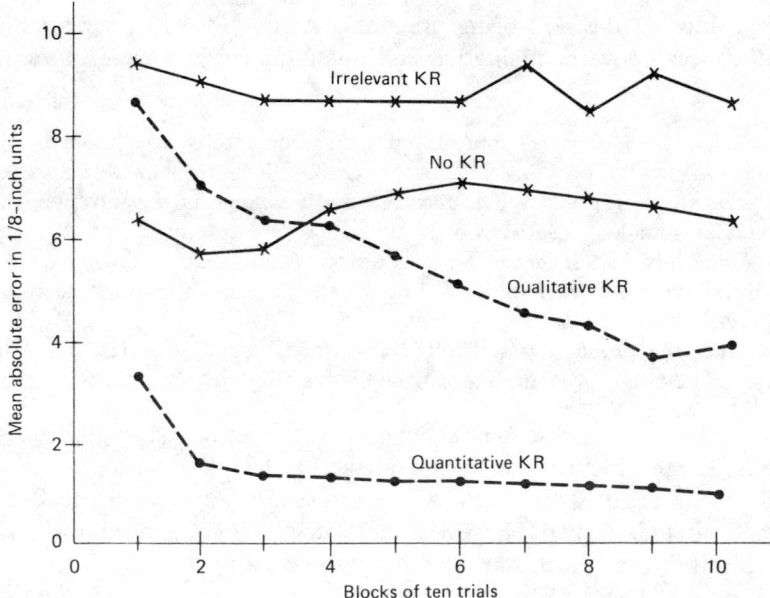

FIGURE 31 Precision of knowledge of results and learning of a line drawing task. (Trowbridge and Cason, 1932. Reprinted from M. H. Trowbridge and H. Cason, An experimental study of Thorndike's theory of learning. *Journal of General Psychology*, 1932, **7**, 245–258, by permission of The Journal Press).

1/4 inch; if he said "minus 4," this represented an undershoot of 1/2 inch. This latter group displayed the greatest improvement over the 100 trials. A fourth group, given a nonsense syllable after every response, showed roughly the same effects as the no-knowledge-of-results group. This was a good control group since any verbal response by the experimenter after each movement might facilitate performance, and thus improvement might have been due to this effect rather than knowledge of results.

These results were duplicated in another study by Bilodeau, Bilodeau, and Schumsky (1959), where they had subjects practice a positioning task for 20 trials. Again, the group that received no knowledge of results did not improve their performance, whereas the knowledge-of-results group improved considerably.

Preciseness of knowledge of results.   When an instructor gives a learner augmented knowledge of results, he is often in a quandary as to how precise he should be. Should he keep his comments general so that the learner can easily understand them, or should he be very precise so that the learner can gain as much knowledge as possible? From the findings of Trowbridge and Cason (1932) presented in Figure 31, one would conclude that the more precise or quantitative knowledge of results can be the better will be the acquisition of the skill being practiced. Adams (1971), in discussing the differences between qualitative and quantitative knowledge of results states:

Theoretically, the finding that more rapid acquisition results from more precise KR follows from the position that motor learning is a problem to be solved. Information in the form of KR is received and a change in the movement on the next trial is made on the basis of it. When, say, the subject is told "Wrong," he has vague information because he is informed only that an error has been made, but he knows neither the direction nor the amount of error. As a result, the correction will tend to be poor each time and the rate of learning will be slow because the problem is difficult. In contrast, quantitative KR gives the direction and amount of error, and learning is faster.

Since there is no research showing that knowledge of results can be too precise, the practical conclusion might be that the teacher or coach should be as precise as possible whenever presenting augmented knowledge of results to the learner. However, there definitely is a need for more research in this area particularly, with the question of how precise knowledge of results should be for different ability levels as well as for different age groups.

Frequency of knowledge of results. Should a teacher or coach give augmented knowledge of results after every attempt at the skill by the learner? In other words, does learning depend on the total number of times knowledge of results are given, or is it sufficient to give them only intermittently? Bilodeau and Bilodeau (1958a) provide some answers to this question in that they give different groups of subjects' knowledge of results after every trial, every third trial, every fourth trial, and every tenth trial. Their task involved how accurately they would turn a knob, and the total number of trials was varied so that all groups received 10 trials. In one part of their results, the authors plotted the performance curves of the four groups for each of the 10 trials immediately following the presentation of knowledge of results. This analysis showed that all groups learned exactly the same amount, indicating that the important issue is the number of times knowledge of results is given, with the actual number of trials with no knowledge of results presented being relatively unimportant. This finding is somewhat similar to those presented earlier, where it was shown that knowledge of results is necessary for learning. Thus, the teacher or coach would be wise to give augmented knowledge of results at relatively frequent intervals.

The timing of knowledge of results. In a learning situation, when a learner receives augmented knowledge of results between two attempts at performing a skill, there are two time gaps that are of considerable importance. The first gap, called the knowledge-of-results delay interval, occurs between the point at which the learner completes the skill and the point at which he receives knowledge of results. For knowledge of results to be effective, presumably the learner must retain in memory the feedback received from performance so that it can be compared with the results achieved. From previous discussions of short-term memory in this book we know that this storage system is limited by time (that is, forgetting increases with time) and attention distractions (that is, if the learner's attention is not on the information in memory, forgetting will be increased), and thus the gap in time becomes important. The second gap of time, called the post-knowledge-of-results delay interval, occurs after knowledge of results is given and before the next movement can be attempted. Here the learner must remember his previous performance as well as the comparison of this performance to the knowledge of results in order that he may modify his motor schema and enhance the likelihood of a successful movement.

At what point in time should knowledge of results be given? If they are given too quickly after the completion of the performance, they may interfere with the organization and consolidation of feedback, from the movement, into memory. On the other hand, if they are delayed too long, the learner's attention may be distracted by events happening around him or by his performing other movements unrelated to the movement to be learned. Similarly, memory processes occurring during the interval between the time when knowledge of results is given and when the next movement is attempted can also be affected by the learner's activities.

The research results are quite clear in indicating that the knowledge-of-results delay interval has relatively little influence on learning efficiency as long as there is no interfering activity between performance and presentation of knowledge of results. Delays of up to an hour (Bilodeau and Bilodeau, 1958b) have been shown not to affect learning when compared with delays as short as 20 or 30 seconds. However, if physical activity in the form of repetitions of the movement takes place between the initial movement and presentation of its knowledge of results, then learning is adversely affected (I. Bilodeau, 1956; Lavery and Suddon, 1962). Thus it would appear that reasonable delays can be tolerated in the knowledge-of-results delay interval, but if possible this interval should be free from interfering activity.

For the postknowledge-of-results delay interval different results have been found. In the only motor learning study done on this topic, Weinberg, Guy, and Tupper (1964) found that for intervals of 1, 5, 10, and 20 seconds the 1-second interval produced poorer performance than the others, with no differences apparent among these latter conditions. The authors' interpretation of these results was that some minimal processing time is needed to process the knowledge-of-results information and compare it with the memory of the completed movement. This processing time was thought to be no longer than 5 seconds. Teachers of motor skills might be wise to have their students spend a small amount of time in organizing their next response after augmented knowledge of results is given.

Summary

The purpose of this chapter was to present a view of how perceptual-motor skills are learned. Since this involves the concept of memory, two learning models that incorporated motor memory into a theoretical framework that accounted for the learning process were described. It was seen that motor memory consisted of various types of information (visual, kinesthetic, efference, knowledge of results), but no exact form of internalization was specified by these models. To gain an understanding of how information in motor memory might be represented, some research in motor short-term memory was discussed. This work showed that motor memory might actually be represented by an image (a nonverbal memory code) that is used as the code for retaining kinesthetic information.

To understand further the nature of motor memory and to determine how movement information is coded the concept of the schema was introduced. The schema was seen as a generalized source of information about movement that organizes information according to rules and principles. It was postulated that the way in which this information was acquired was through the establishment of intersensory equivalence among the various sensory systems that are used to process movement-related information. This store of highly integrated information was, in effect, seen as a schema capable of producing unique motor programs (schema instances) that were matched to specific environmental demands. In this regard it was noted that the concept of motor programs that entailed storing highly rigid sequences of motor commands for use in specific situations was not only unnecessary but actually an inefficient way of obtaining highly skilled behavior. Finally, since the development of motor schemata was seen to be heavily dependent on a learner receiving knowledge of results and performance, the literature dealing with the known principles of these types of feedback was reviewed.

Suggested Readings

Performance Models That Incorporate the "Motor" Permanent Store

Adams, J. A., A closed-loop theory of motor learning. *Journal of Motor Behavior*, 1971, **3,** 111–150.

Chase, R. A., An information-flow model of the organization of motor activity. Part I: Transduction, transmission, and central control of sensory information. *Journal of Nervous and Mental Disease*, 1965a, **140,** 239–251.

Chase, R. A., An information-flow model of the organization of motor activity. Part II: Sampling, central processing, and utilization of sensory information. *Journal of Nervous and Mental Disease*, 1965b, **140,** 334–350.

Crossman, E. R. F. W., Information processes in human skill. *British Medical Bulletin*, 1964, **20,** 32–37.

Laszlo, Judith I., and Bairstow, P. J., Accuracy of movement, peripheral feedback and efference copy. *Journal of Motor Behavior*, 1971, **3,** 241–252.

Pew, R. W., Levels of analysis in motor control. *Brain Research*, 1974, **71,** 393–400.

Schmidt, R. A., *Motor Skills*. New York: Harper & Row, 1975.

Short-Term Motor Memory in Learning

Bartlett, F. C., *Remembering: A Study in Experimental and Social Psychology*. New York: Cambridge, 1961.

Keele, S. W., *Attention and Human Performance*. Pacific Palisades, Calif.: Goodyear, 1973.

Posner, M. I., Short term memory systems in human information processing. In R. N. Haber (Ed.), *Information-Processing Approaches to Visual Perceptions*. New York: Holt, Rinehart and Winston, 1969.

The Schema as Motor Memory

Bartlett, F. C., *Remembering: A Study in Experimental and Social Psychology*. New York: Cambridge, 1961.

Pew, R. W., Levels of analysis in motor control. *Brain Research*, 1974, **71,** 393–400.

Schmidt, R. A., *Motor Skills*. New York: Harper & Row, 1975.

Knowledge of Results and Performance

Adams, J. A., A closed-loop theory of motor learning. *Journal of Motor Behavior*, 1971, **3,** 111–150.

Bilodeau, E. A. (Ed.), *Principles of Skill Acquisition*. New York: Academic Press, 1969.

Holding, D. H., *Principles of Training*. New York: Pergamon, 1965.

Section 4

Applications and Implications

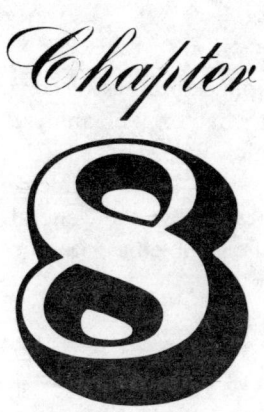

Chapter 8

Applications of the Information Processing Model to Motor Performance and Learning Problems

Introduction

The previous seven chapters of this book were concerned with establishing a basic framework by which perceptual motor performance and learning could be conceptualized. A serious student should now have enough information to enable him to analyze any perceptual-motor activity in terms of its underlying processes. It should be emphasized, however, that the component human performance model presented in this book should only be considered a guide to conceptualizing those processes underlying the successful performance and learning of physical activity. The important point is that if students interested in studying physical activity apply the human performance model to coaching, teaching, or research problems, they should do so with the intent of seeing whether the model is adequate for their purposes. If not, it is hoped that the result will be a creative adaptation of the model that will more resemble the particular aspects of the problem. The serious student will then attempt to verify whether his modified model is more effective than the original one. Through this process knowledge about human performance and learning will be increased, and greater benefits can be derived through its various applications.

To demonstrate how the principles of the human performance model, as established in the first seven chapters, might be applied to areas of concern to the student of physical activity, the present chapter will analyze several pertinent motor performance and learning topics. The reader might immediately be able to apply the results of this analysis to some problem, but the intent, as stated before, will be to demonstrate how the general human performance model can be applied to specific problems with the hope of stimulating creative thought in these areas.

A Teaching Model

Since teaching is a complex phenomenon, which entails applying countless principles of performance and learning to the teaching situation, a teaching model will be presented that outlines six broad components of behavior that are central to learning and thus illustrate the more important principles a teacher should be intimately familiar with. Figure 32 schematically displays these components of behavior.

Each of the components of this teaching model will be later described in detail; however, a brief overview of the model will be presented here. Figure 32 depicts two broad divisions of behavior. The first deals with the state of the individual in terms of his readiness and willingness to receive and process information. This motivation and alertness dimension is crucial to the learning process in that if a learner is not alert and motivated to learn, the teaching process will be unsuccessful no matter how well structured it is.

The other dimension of behavior, as depicted in Figure 32, deals with aspects of behavior closely aligned to the concept of the learner as an information processor and, as such, depicts information processes that have been discussed in previous chapters of this book. Central to the development of efficient information processes is the establishment, in the learner, of well-defined goals of performance. These goals not only influence how a learner will formulate a plan of action but, to a degree, also affect the selection of input information that will be processed by the performer's limited capacity information processing system. Although the goals may partly influence the selective attention process, there are also other factors that are crucial to the efficient selection of information from the learner's environment and feedback, and these will be discussed later. By knowing the goals of the performance and by selectively attending to the teacher's instructions and demonstrations, the learner then formulates a plan for action that not only specifies the components of the movement, as well as their sequential and temporal organization, but also specifies how this movement must be integrated with the specific environmental situation confronted by the learner. Thus both environmental and move-

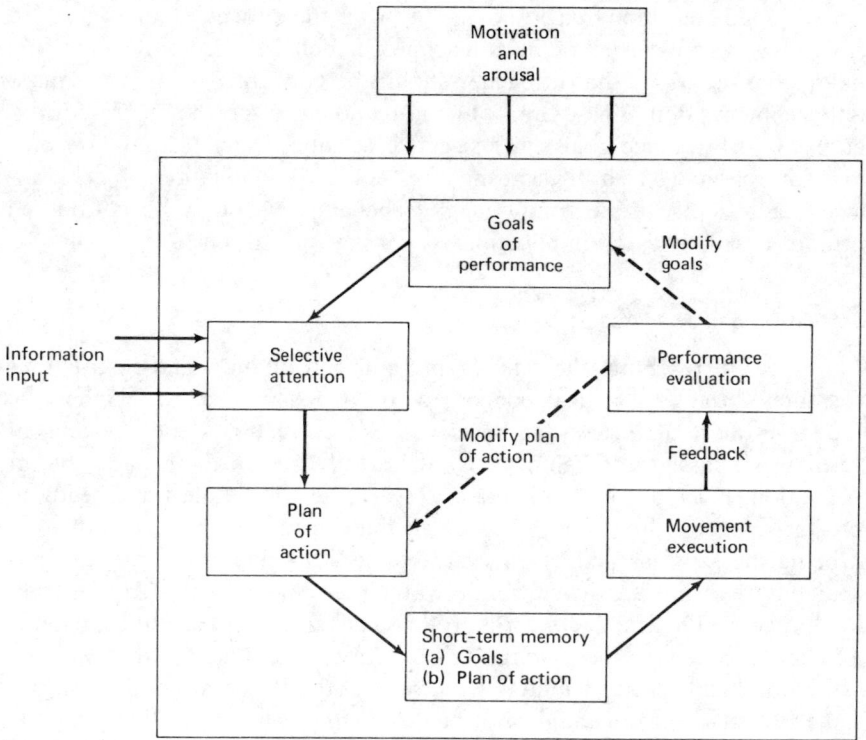

FIGURE 32 A model depicting the performance and learning components of teaching.

ment cues must be integrated into a plan for action. This information, if it is to be remembered for any length of time, must then be stored in memory. Thus the next crucial consideration in the instruction process has to do with the factors that influence the retention of this information. Figure 32 depicts this component as short-term memory.

Once the learner acquires sufficient information for the plan of action, the movement is then executed and the learner receives feedback from his attempt. Through the use of this feedback the learner evaluates his performance and determines the adequacy of his original goal and/or plan of action. If either or both are inadequate, modifications to one or both of these processes are made and the learner again attempts the movement. Through repetition of this sequence, performance is slowly modified so that it becomes more efficient and appropriate to the requirements of the situation.

As stated earlier, if a teacher becomes familiar with the processes depicted in Figure 32, a number of implications for instruction will become immediately apparent, and in this way the processes in Figure 32 can really be conceived of in a teaching model. In effect, there are six major considerations that a teacher should be concerned with when planning for instruction. These are: (1) motivation and alertness; (2) formulation of performance goals; (3) selective attention; (4) formulation of a plan for action; (5) short-term memory; and (6) evaluation of performance. Each one of these components of behavior will now be considered in more detail, and the implications for instruction discussed.

Motivation and Alertness

Since, in teaching, the teacher presents information and instructions to students, the first critical concern of the teacher must be whether the student is alert and ready to receive this information. The concept of alertness, discussed in Chapter 3, is intrinsically tied to the broad topic of motivation. If a student is motivated to learn, he will be alert and ready to receive pertinent information. If we can think of alertness and motivation as being the same as activation (as discussed in Chapter 3), we can immediately see what a teacher can do to facilitate this aspect of the instruction process. The chief concern of the teacher is to keep the students optimally aroused. In the long run this is probably best achieved by making instructions and teaching material relevant to the interests and aspirations of the students. When dealing with the teaching of physical activity, a good teacher will spend some time determining what relevance this material has for the students. Some students may simply want instruction so that their performance will be enhanced; others may want physical activity for health reasons and the teacher may want to spend some time on explaining how physical activity contributes to a healthful life style. In addition to these more immediate goals, the teacher may also have an educational philosophy that he wants to impart to the students, and it may require a shaping of students' interests and aspirations over a longer period of time.

Although the above points are important for the maintenance of long-range motivation, other devices are open to the teacher to create alertness over shorter periods of time. A pleasing voice that varies in intensity is one such device. The judicious use of challenging situations is another.

According to activation theory, an important point to be kept in mind is that individual differences occur in terms of the optimal level of arousal for performance and learning. A teacher should be aware of the different personality types that predispose a student to the ways in which he reacts to increased arousal. Some students may require little arousal increase to reach this optimal point, whereas others may have to be under conditions that are designed to increase arousal greatly in order for them to reach their optimal level.

Formulation of the Goals of Performance

The goal of a particular perceptual-motor skill is to reduce a discrepancy between the state of a particular environmental situation and the state that an individual, considering his needs and desires, wishes the environment to be in. The performer resolves this discrepancy by producing a movement with a particular outcome that was planned to change the environment. Thus, before he can plan an effective movement, the goal must be perfectly clear. While for most learners the goal is rather apparent (for example, put the ball in the basket; hit the ball; jump over the bar), these are global goals and the teacher must appreciate that skills that constitute complicated games or activities might each have subgoals that contribute, either immediately or in the long run, to the global goal. For example, the global goal of a badminton player is to hit the bird in such a way that his opponent cannot return it. However, the goal of a clear in badminton, while eventually contributing to the former goal, is different in that it usually has the purpose of forcing a weak return so that the next stroke can be offensive in nature. The point, then, is that a teacher must ensure not only that the overall goal of an activity is apparent, but also that the goals of the skills that make up a complex activity are also perfectly clear. If these goals are not clear, confusion will result and effective plans of action will not be made.

In addition to the influence that well-defined goals of performance can have on the formation of plans of action, the goals will also affect, to some degree, what general sources of information a learner will attend to. An instructor, by defining the goals of the skill, will cause the learner to narrow his attention to a particular class of events pertinent to the successful accomplishment of the goals. These events will consist of environmental situations that the movement is performed in as well as what the pertinent movement characteristics of a successful movement are. However, this environmental and movement information should be described only in general terms at this stage in the teaching model so that the learner receives a good overall impression of what the goals of performance are. Detailed knowledge about appropriate or pertinent environmental and movement information should be given in later stages of the instructional sequence as outlined below.

Selective Attention

Being alert and motivated and knowing the global goals of performance do not necessarily imply that a student will correctly interpret the instructions and descriptions provided by the teacher or will be able to attend to the specific environmental movement cues leading to successful performance. Knowing what to attend to involves the phenomenon of selective attention, which was dealt with at length in Chapter 4. Of fundamental concern to the teacher, in regard to considering how selective attention influences teaching, are the issues of establishing pertinence and realizing the limitations imposed on the performer by the selective attention process.

As established in Chapter 4, when Norman's (1969) model of selective attention was discussed, an important aspect of selective attention is the role that expectations and contextual cues play in establishing pertinence for the performer. In essence, this implies that an individual who knows what is about to happen will be able to attend to relevant incoming information selectively and thus facilitate his information processing ability. The fact that pertinence, in practical terms, can be equated with past experience implies that a teacher can manipulate an individual's selective attention either by providing him with the experience that would establish pertinence or by pointing out how his already established past experiences are relevant to the performance of the to-be-learned skill. The importance of establishing pertinence was discussed at length in Chapter 4, and it cannot be overemphasized here that this is a crucial issue in instructional methodology. A learner must know, through pertinence, what to attend to or the learning process will be impeded by his attending to irrelevant information.

Related to the concept of pertinence is the limitation placed on processing information by the act of selectively attending to some input. Selective attention requires central processing capacity and, as a result, while an individual selectively attends to one source of information all other sources of information are at least temporarily blocked out. In turn, the less well developed an individual's pertinence is, the greater the limitation imposed by the selective attention process. In other words, those individuals who have very few expectations (that is, anticipations and predictions) or are able to make use of only small amounts of contextual information are severely limited by the selective attention process. They can selectively attend to only one thing at a time and, since they lack the ability to predict into the future, each incoming piece of information must be processed individually, and thus a great demand is made on the central processing capacity.

The above two issues, pertinence and a limited capacity to selectively attend to incoming information when pertinence has not been fully established, have direct implications for the teaching of inexperienced performers. First, the teacher must always attempt to give the learner some prior information about the skill so that he knows what to expect while he performs it. Second, since selective attention places a demand on the cen-

Applications of the Information Processing Model to Motor Performance

tral processing capacity, the instructor not only must provide pertinence but also must restrict the total number of events that he wants the performer to attend to. This is especially so in the very early stages of learning. A naive performer will be able to attend to only one source of information at a time; if the instructor tries to have him attend to two sources simultaneously, one source will be ignored. This implies that the teacher will have to make a thorough task analysis, where analysis is made of the components of the task, the cues of most relevance for the learner's stage of performance, and the types and numbers of instructions or cues that should be made available to the learner.

A practical example of this latter point is teaching the basketball dribble to naive performers. Ideally, good basketball players very rarely have to attend to the act of controlling the ball while dribbling. Their attention is usually focused on the strategy of the game. However, to a naive performer, attending to the feedback received from bouncing a ball occupies a good deal of his central processing capacity and if a teacher instructs him to attend to other things as well, such as the position of his teammates or opponents, more than likely he will perform the dribble poorly. Thus, it may be wise to start the skill of dribbling by having the performer practice under instructions that focus his attention on the relevant information (feedback) necessary to control the ball. Once this skill is developed (that is, the individual has established pertinence for this type of information, which makes it somewhat redundant) the instructor can then introduce the next most relevant information that must be attended to for proper dribbling ability.

Relevant information and instructional sets. Implied in the above discussion is the ability of the teacher to direct the learner's attention, by establishing pertinence, to relevant sources of information. It must be appreciated that for the performance of any skill there is a large amount of information available to the performer, some of which is relevant and much of which is irrelevant to the successful performance of that skill. A teacher's instructions and demonstrations should be carefully planned so as to aid the performer in distinguishing between these two sources of information. To establish pertinence for relevant sources of information the teacher must use instructional sets to guide a learner's performance. Generally speaking, there are two major types of instructional sets with which the teacher should be concerned. First, there are instructional sets for establishing pertinence for relevant information arising from the environment the learner performs in. For open skills, the teacher must attempt to aid the learner in interpreting relevant sources of information that will successfully guide the performance of the skill. Here, pointing out cues that will aid anticipation or prediction of events would be most valuable. For closed skills, the teacher should emphasize attention to those relevant environmental cues that a performer can refer to as he performs the skill.

The second major type of instructional set that a teacher can utilize is the instructional set for feedback arising from the performance of the skill. As will be pointed out in a later part of this teaching model, an important aspect of skill learning is the evaluation of the success of movement. This evaluation is critically dependent on the use of feedback in that it must be compared to what the individual intended to do. However, before feedback can be used for this evaluation process, it must be selectively attended to and thus, for this reason, can be treated in a manner similar to how environmental information is selectively attended to. In other words, there are relevant and irrelevant sources of feedback information, and to enhance the learning process the teacher must direct the learner's attention to the relevant feedback cues. One effective way of doing this is through the use of instructional sets for feedback, whereby a teacher instructs a performer, before he attempts a skill, to attend to a particular source of feedback. In this way a performer's ability to evaluate the success of his performance is enhanced.

Formulation of the Plan for Action

The above description of how selective attention limits a learner's information processing ability has direct implications for how well a teacher can develop, within the learner, a plan for action. Before any movement can be performed by the learner he must first take into consideration the characteristics of the environment in which the movement will be executed. Thus the teacher will be required to make the learner aware of the relevant environmental cues with which the execution of the movement must be matched. Second, and just as important, the teacher must also specify the various components of the movement, as well as their temporal and spatial organization. The ability to plan a movement in this way is directly dependent upon the success of an individual in generating a unique schema instance, as discussed in Chapter 7.

It is proposed that a teacher can best facilitate the development of a plan for action by considering the principles discussed in Chapters 6 and 7 in regard to the hierarchical and sequential organization of perceptual-motor skills, the concept of the computer analogy, and the concept of the idea or image of a skill. The first consideration is to give the student an overall plan or idea of the movement that will guide the execution of the components. This plan should be able to be derived from the learner's past experiences in movement (that is, the schema for movement) and, in essence, involves the concept of transfer of learning (to be discussed in a later section of this chapter). This also implies, of course, that the instructions of a teacher will be at a level appropriate to the learner's level of past experience. Through this process, then, the resulting executive program specifies not only the various components of the movement but also the movement's hierarchical and sequential organization. The important issue in treating a motor plan in this way is that it stresses the principle of hierarchical and sequential organization and introduces the idea (executive program) that a movement has control over the components of the movement. Both the idea and the components of the movement must be clear to the performer so that he can compare, through the use of feedback, the outcome of the movement (that is, the execution of the components) with the idea, or overall plan, of the movement. This process is vital to the learning of skills and will be covered in more detail below.

Short-Term Memory

The next consideration involved in most aspects of the instructional process concerns the characteristics of short-term memory. To this point the teaching model has described the importance of establishing goals for performance, directing the learner's attention to important environmental cues, and directing his attention to the movement components necessary to execute the movement. Presumably, all this has occurred in an instructional situation where the teacher has verbally presented several points and perhaps demonstrated the to-be-learned movement. Even if the learner has been able to selectively attend to these instructions and demonstrations there is still the question of whether he will be able to remember them. Thus, of major concern to the teacher at this point in the instruction process is how a student stores information in short-term memory; what factors enhance this storage, and what influences the passage of this information from short-term memory to a more stable and enduring long-term memory. These processes can be described under the following general headings: (1) coding of information; (2) capacity of short-term memory; and (3) retention characteristics of short-term memory.

Coding of information. As was pointed out in Chapter 7, not much is known about how movement-related information is stored in short-term memory. If we did have a complete picture of how a learner represents movement in memory, the instructor could facilitate the instruction process by organizing and presenting instructions and demonstrations in a form compatible with that found in memory. In this way the transformation process (that is, transforming an instruction or demonstration into a memory form) would be greatly simplified and would result in better storage. In a similar way the instructor could also provide the student with learning sets for receiving feedback of movement that would facilitate the transformation of this feedback into memory.

The basic purpose of instruction is to give the performer a clear idea of what he must do, and also to give him a method of evaluating whether what he did was what he intended to do. This obviously involves, as was shown in Chapter 7, the formation of an image or standard movement as well as a means of comparing feedback to the image. What is the form of memory representation of this image? Although it is by no means clear, the discussion in Chapter 7 indicated that vision appears to be a vital component. It seems that proprioceptive information must be combined with visual information in order for a clear image to be developed. Thus the teacher almost always should attempt to present instructions or ideas in a visual form through the judicious use of demonstrations, film loops, and video tape replays. Adams (1971) also suggests that early perceptual-motor learning has a large verbal component to it. This indicates that the image may also have a verbal component to it. Perhaps the verbalization of the requirements of a skill (many learners do this automatically) is the first step in establishing a visual image of the skill. Thus having students explain verbally what they are to do as well as giving them rich and varied visual information most likely will lead to an efficient coding of information in short-term memory. This, however, is somewhat speculative and must await further research evidence before becoming a valid technique in the instruction process.

Capacity of short-term memory. Whether a teacher is giving instructions, demonstrations, or augmented feedback, he must always keep in mind the capacity of the learner for retaining a number of items in memory. For naive performers this capacity is very low and generally speaking a teacher should not expect students to retain more than two or three items for any length of time. The general principle would be that the fewer number of items (instructions, descriptions, feedback cues) presented, the better they will be remembered. However, once a student has gained some experience in a skill, the teacher can use this as a base to increase the detail of his instructions or demonstrations. However, it would appear from the research literature that there should never be more than about seven items presented at any given time to an individual. Seven items appears to be a capacity for short-term memory above which information is automatically lost from memory.

An important instructional method that a teacher can use to overcome this apparent capacity is to use descriptive phrases that "chunk" items together into larger meaningful units. Chunking was defined and discussed in Chapter 4, and it is suggested here that this is a powerful tool for instructional purposes. For instance, when giving detailed instructions on the position and action of the hand in dribbling a basketball, a teacher can easily exceed the capacity of short-term memory. However, if he can chunk these details under a descriptor phrase like "fingertip control," the learner is able to associate and organize the specific facts of ball control under this phrase. As a result, because the information is organized, the load on memory is lessened and the chances of retaining the complete description is increased. Likewise, when explaining the overhead clear in badminton, two important aspects of this skill are the position of the racket as it is brought back in preparation to hitting the shuttlecock and the action of the racket as it goes from this position to the point of contact with the shuttlecock. Obviously a teacher can give a detailed explanation of both these components and greatly exceed a learner's short-term memory capacity. If instead, these two components can be likened to "scratching your back" and "throwing the racket (similar to throwing a ball) to the ceiling," the memory load is greatly decreased in that these two phrases trigger off images that are appropriate for the correct performance of the clear.

The point of the above discussion, then, is that through imaginative phrases and instructions a teacher can greatly enhance the probability that students will retain critical aspects of the skill. The use of such techniques is necessitated by the inherent limitation imposed upon a performer by his short-term memory capacity.

Retention characteristics of short-term memory. Once the teacher has presented information to the student regarding the skill to be learned his next concern is with attempting to ensure that it will not be forgotten. As mentioned in Chapter 1, new material in short-term memory is very susceptible to forgetting, especially for about the first 60 seconds after presentation of the to-be-learned material. For purposes of teaching, there are three main characteristics of short-term memory that a teacher should be knowledgeable about so that he can facilitate the retention of information and, in essence, ensure its passage to a more permanent type of long-term memory. These are: (1) attention and rehearsal; (2) time between presentation and recall; and (3) interference.

After information enters short-term memory, its retention is dependent upon the student's ability to maintain attention on the to-be-remembered material. If his attention is used for other purposes, the material in memory begins to be forgotten, with most of the forgetting occurring in about the first 60 seconds that attention is not on the material. To facilitate retention and retard the forgetting process the teacher must attempt to keep the student's attention on the material. The most obvious way for doing this when teaching a perceptual-motor skill is to have the student perform the skill as soon as possible after initial instructions and demonstrations have been presented. This represents overt rehearsal and ensures that the student is thinking about the skill. Like overt repetition of some verbal material, the more times a movement is practiced the more likely it will be passed on to long-term memory. Thus, initially it is important to keep attention on the to-be-remembered material by planning for as many repetitions as possible.

Another possibility for rehearsal of motor skills, especially in the early phase of learning, occurs when students are asked to verbally repeat the requirements of the skill, either overtly or covertly. This is a form of mental practice and would surely help instructions or instructional sets to become fixed in memory through repetition. This type of rehearsal can occur through the use of summaries by the teacher at the end of an instructional period and also by the teacher's questioning students as to what they thought the essential points of the instructional period were. Review periods at the beginning of each lesson would also serve the same function. However, the teacher should keep in mind that in order to ensure that a student's attention is on the review material, a wise technique will be to ask the student to recall the essential point of the previous lesson rather than just have the teacher present a review to, perhaps, an inattentive audience.

The second major consideration for a teacher attempting to facilitate memory of perceptual-motor skills is the time between presentation and recall of the to-be-remembered material. There will inevitably be a delay between presentation of instructions for a perceptual-motor skill and the performance of that skill. During this time it is most certain that a student's attention will not always be on the skill, and therefore forgetting will occur. For this reason an instructor must minimize, as much as possible, the time between presentation of instructions and performance. When dealing with groups of students it is imperative that each student perform the skill as soon as possible. Therefore the teacher must avoid long lineups in which a student must wait his turn for a considerable time. In essence, the teacher must plan for as much involvement from as many students as possible. This should be an important consideration in any lesson plan.

The last consideration for facilitating retention of information in short-term memory deals with the concept of interference. When information is stored in short-term memory, it can be interfered with in two ways. First, as already mentioned, the student's attention can be taken away from the material and, because of a lack of rehearsal, it will be forgotten. Second, the activity that causes the attention to be taken away can directly interfere with the representation in memory of the to-be-remembered material. In other words, there is a double cause of potential forgetting. While not much is known about what kind of activity directly interferes with the memory of perceptual-motor skills, it is safe to say that a teacher should keep all unrelated activity to a minimum during the student's first several attempts at learning a new skill. Other skills should not be introduced until the learner has a good grasp of the basic idea of the new skill.

Performance Evaluation and Feedback

After formulating a plan for action and having it in memory, the performer must now attempt the movement. After the execution, if learning is to occur, he must then evaluate the movement to determine not only whether the movement was executed properly but also whether the movement accomplished the original goal. This evaluation process is fundamental to learning and can be influenced greatly by the teacher through instructional methodology. Of initial concern to this evaluation process is the ability of the learner to process feedback. Feedback, used here in its broadest sense, can be considered as another input variable to the limited capacity information processing system, and therefore the limitation imposed by selective attention and short-term memory apply to this variable as well. One can now appreciate the complexity of the learning process from the viewpoint of the performer as well as of the teacher. Instructions and demonstrations must be presented and remembered, relevant environmental cues must be considered, an idea of the movement must be generated, and a plan of action must be formulated and executed. All of these aspects must be attended to and remembered. If we add to this, now, the necessity for attending to and remembering pertinent aspects of the feedback from the execution of the skill, there is little wonder that learning a new skill takes a relatively long time. There remains little doubt that a teacher must have a good understanding of the selective attention and short-term memory capacities of performers if he is to formulate instructional methodologies designed to facilitate learning.

Although Figure 32 depicted modification of the goals of performance and the plan for action through the use of dotted lines, space in that schematic diagram did not permit full details of how feedback is used. Figure 33 thus presents a more detailed illustration of this process. Any feedback received by the performer, whether it be knowledge of results (KR) or knowledge of performance (KP) from his own actions or from a teacher, faces the same limitation due to selective attention as any other input information. That is, it must be selectively attended to if it is to have access to the limited capacity information processing system. Once it is selectively attended to, it then enters memory, where the original goals of performance and plan of action should also be stored. Thus, as indicated in Figure 33, if a teacher has provided effective instructions in the form of descriptions and instructional sets, the learner, after completing an attempt at a movement, should have in his short-term memory four types of information: (1) the original goal of the movement; (2) the outcome of

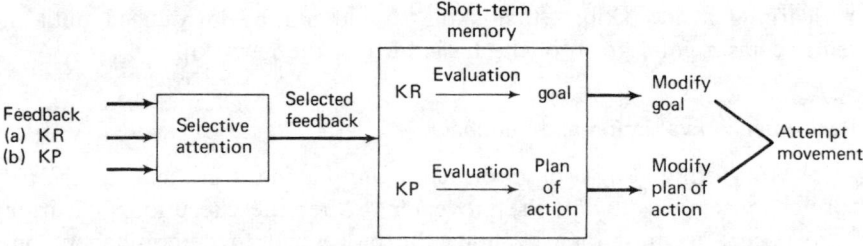

FIGURE 33 An illustration of how KR & KP are used to modify the goal and the plan of action of a to-be-learned movement.

the movement; (3) the image and the plan for action; and (4) the actual way in which the movement was executed. These sources of information are not necessarily the same since the goal and the outcome of the movement may or may not coincide and, as well, the way in which a movement was performed may not correspond with the initial image or plan of action.

With these four sources of information in short-term memory the learner is now able to make the necessary evaluation of his performance. The end result should be a modification of the original goal and/or plan of action in an attempt to make the movement more successful in the next attempt. Through repeated attempts, after each of which there occurs an evaluation and modification, the movement will become increasingly effective; that is, there are observed increments in performance due to the learning process.

As a guide to this evaluation process the teacher should consider the use of the decision matrix presented in Figure 30 in Chapter 7. If the teacher can ensure that this type of evaluation process can occur each time a learner performs a movement, learning will be enhanced. As indicated in Chapter 7, in the discussion of Figure 30, the evaluation of movement is dependent upon ability of the learner to receive both knowledge of results and performance. Although the instructor can aid the learner in attending to this information through instructional sets, it may be that the learner is still unable to perceive the relevant feedback. In this case the teacher should be prepared to give augmented knowledge of performance and results to facilitate the learner's evaluation process. When this is done, it is important to remember that these two types of information are not the same (one is knowledge of outcome and the other is knowledge of movement) and that both contribute separately and in combination to the evaluation process. A teacher must therefore evaluate a learner's performance to determine exactly what kind of augmented feedback is necessary. Once this is accomplished, the teacher must then remember to keep the limitations of selective attention and short-term memory in mind as he presents the augmented feedback to the learner. In particular, after a learner attempts a movement, it will be wise for the teacher not to give augmented feedback for at least a few moments. Right after a skill has been performed, the learner must have his attention on selectively attending to and coding the relevant feedback information, and any interruption of this process by the teacher in giving augmented feedback will result in immediate forgetting.

Since this section on performance evaluation and feedback is very important, a short step-by-step summary of the more important considerations will be presented.

1. Evaluation of movement, which leads to modification of future attempts and thus learning, involves using knowledge of results and performance in comparison with the goal and the plan of action.
2. All four of the above types of information are dependent on short-term memory in that they must be retained over periods of time.
3. Selective attention is an important factor in determining how well these sources of information enter memory.
4. Instructional sets can facilitate the reception of feedback, and therefore are a necessary part of instructional methodology.
5. Oftentimes a learner will not be able to perceive the relevant feedback from his actions and the teacher will have to provide augmented feedback.
6. The learner should be encouraged to evaluate his own movement, and thus the teacher should provide uninterrupted time after each movement execution, during which feedback from the movement can be coded into memory and the complex evaluation process can occur without the learner's attention being distracted.
7. The teacher must appreciate the separate and combined roles that knowledge of results and performance play in the learning of perceptual-motor skills in terms of how they are used in the evaluation of performance and subsequent modification of the goal and plan for action.

The Teaching Model and Phases of Skill Learning

The immediately preceding section has presented a general teaching model as a guide for instruction. However, before this model can be effectively applied, consideration must be given to how a teacher should modify his instructions, demonstrations, use of feedback, and so on, to take into account differences in students' initial skill levels. Undoubtedly a teacher will approach the instruction of complete novices much differently than instruction of a group of relatively skilled individuals. The characteristics of learners at different phases of learning and the implications these differences have for instruction comprise the topic of this section.

One characteristic of performers at specific phases of learning is that they may use different types of feedback in the planning, execution, and evaluation of this performance. One study that demonstrates the principle that different phases of learning are dependent on different types of feedback is one made by Fleishman and Rich (1963), who investigated the roles of kinesthesis and spatial orientations in learning a two-hand coordination task. This perceptual-motor task required the subject to follow a disk, moving at irregular rates around a circle, with a spot controlled by rotating two handles, one with each hand. One hand controlled the handle that moved the spot toward and away from the subject's body, while the other hand controlled the movement of the spot from left to right. All subjects were given 40 one-minute trials on this task.

In addition to performing the two-hand coordination task, the subjects were tested on their kinesthetic and spatial sensitivity abilities. The subjects were then divided into the best 20 and the worst 20 on spatial sensitivity and the best 20 and worst 20 on kinesthetic sensitivity.

The results showed that those 20 subjects with the best spatial sensitivity performed better, early in learning, than those with the worst spatial sensitivity, thus indicating, perhaps, that the use of visual information is most important at this stage of practice. However, at the end of the 40 trials the fact that there was virtually no difference between these two groups suggested that late in learning the role of visual information is not that important.

Almost the exact reverse of these results was obtained when the performance characteristics of the best and worst subjects in kinesthetic sensitivity was examined. Early in learning there was no difference in performance between these two groups, but late in learning those subjects high in kinesthetic sensitivity were superior. These results thus indicated that the ability to use kinesthetic information early in learning is relatively unimportant as when compared to this ability late in learning. More important, the overall results of this study suggest that early in learning the ability to use visual information is very important, but performance late in learning is more dependent on the ability to use kinesthetic information.

The implications of the above study for the understanding of how feedback is used in different phases of learning are that the teacher or coach must be sensitive to what basic types of feedback a learner is using so that the teacher can direct the learner's attention toward the appropriate source of information. For instance, if the findings of Fleishman and Rich's study are valid, the instructor may want to direct the learner's attention toward visual feedback early in the learning of a particular skill. Similarly, any augmented knowledge of results or performance should be phrased in terms of visual information. The important point is that the teacher or coach must be aware of the different phases of learning so that proper use of feedback, relevant to a particular phase, can be employed.

Although the above example serves to illustrate one way in which the characteristics of performance differ as learning level changes, it will be more beneficial to outline in some systematic fashion what is thought to be the number of different learning phases an individual progresses through as he learns a skill. Fitts (1964) has postulated three phases of learning that are ideally suited for this purpose. Moreover, various implications for instruction can be illustrated for each phase. The phases are: (1) the cognitive phase; (2) the associative phase; and (3) the autonomous phase. In describing these phases Fitts made use of terminology utilized in the computer analogy of skills that was covered in Chapter 6 of this book. In this analogy he used the executive program to mean the performer's overall idea of the skill, and subroutines stood for the components of the skill that were grouped hierarchically and sequentially under the executive program. To be consistent with terminology that was introduced in Chapter 7, the schema will now be used in place of executive program, and the schema instance (the plan for action) will indicate a collection of specific subroutines or components that must be executed in a sequential manner with the correct temporal organization in order for the skill to be performed properly.

The Cognitive Phase

According to Fitts, the cognitive phase of learning is concerned with developing within the learner the motor schema of the skill to be learned. In other words, the learner must form an idea of the entire skill, and thus this stage is more cognitive than motor in nature. Except in the very young, under the age of six years, Fitts and Posner (1967) believe that all children possess the necessary movement experiences for learning all new motor skills, and during this first phase of learning the learner must be able to group these experiences together cognitively in a unique fashion to produce the new motor schema. The new schema is really a patchwork of existing movement experiences, all collected from previous motor schemas and cognitively held together to form the basis of a new skill.

Included in the idea of the skill at this phase of learning are the relevant environmental cues that control or regulate the movement. In other words, the learner not only must have an idea of the movement involved but also must be able to recognize and process those cues in the environment to which the movement must be matched. For closed skills this may represent a relatively simple approach for this initial phase of learning. However, for open skills the problem is somewhat more complex in that the environment is constantly changing, and in many cases cues exhibit sequential dependencies that enable prediction or anticipation of events.

Evidence has already been presented (the Fleishman and Rich study) to indicate that visual cues might play a dominant organizing factor in the formation of a new motor schema. Adams (1971) has argued that perceptual-motor skills, early in learning, rely greatly on verbal skills. He takes as evidence for the use of verbal abilities in the formation of motor schemas the fact that learners are highly prone to verbalize the skill they are attempting to acquire. In essence, verbalization of the requirements of a skill may serve to help organize the motor schema as well as permit important environmental cues to be remembered. From this viewpoint it would appear that conceptual or mental development of the requirements of a skill plays an important role in the early acquisition of that skill.

Depending on the complexity of the new skill, this phase may last from only several minutes to a few hours (Fitts, 1964). However, once the individual performs a rough approximation to the desired outcome, he can be considered to have acquired the idea of the skill and he then progresses to the second phase of learning.

Transfer of learned behavior. Since this phase is primarily concerned with establishing an idea of the new skill the teacher should direct all his instructions and demonstrations towards this goal. It is here where the instructor must make full use of the learner's past experience by expressing the new skill in terms of already acquired concepts of movements. In essence, a teacher should plan for the transfer of learning where what is actually transferred are concepts and symbolic behavior derived from the learner's past experience. If the teacher can succeed in making a learner see the similarity between already acquired skills and a new skill this will facilitate the formation of an initial motor schema for the new skill. An example of this principle would be comparing the action of the back swing and forward swing in the overhead clear in badminton to the action involved in throwing a ball. Since throwing is familiar to most individuals, this established concept can be readily transferred to the new skill.

Structuring the environment. Another important consideration that a teacher must make, when dealing with learners at this phase of learning, concerns how he should structure the environment for practice of the to-be-learned movement. Careful thought should be given to those cues in the environment that are relevant to the new skill and thus, keeping in mind the limitations of selective attention and short-term memory, the teacher should first structure the environment as simply as possible. For open skills this may mean using cues or situations that occur most frequently and that are absolutely necessary for the execution of the new skill. Thus the teacher would allow the learner to initially practice under these conditions before introducing less frequently appearing cues or situations. For closed skills the teacher may initially direct the learner's attention to the most important constant relevant cue and once the learner is able to easily attend to this cue, introduce other relevant ones.

Conclusions. In the cognitive phase of learning the emphasis of the instructor should be placed on giving the learner an idea or concept of the movement. As discussed above, the teacher should attempt to keep instruction as simple as possible, highly visual and verbal in nature, and plan for transfer of learned behavior. Once the idea of the skill is achieved, practice in a rather simplified environment should take place. When a learner is able to roughly accomplish the goal of the new skill as well as approximately execute the movement as planned, he can thus be considered to have passed from the first to the second phase of learning.

The Associative Phase

This phase of learning is concerned with: (1) making the schema more exact and integrated; and (2) learning to generate and execute schema instances that match the exact demands of the skill. Schema modification takes place through feedback processes that have already been discussed in this chapter. Although it has not been established by research, one might assume that dependency on visual and verbal information in the formation of the schema is slowly shifted to more dependency on proprioceptive information during this phase.

While the schema becomes more integrated and detailed, the learner must also learn to generate instances of this schema that fit the exact demands of the skill. At first this will be a difficult and slow process, for there are very many possible variations of the components of a skill and the correct hierarchical and sequential order may be hard to achieve. For this reason, errors of movement may involve such things as the wrong sequence of components, the occurrence of an inappropriate component in a sequence, or the wrong timing of the various components in a sequence.

Through learning, however, the individual becomes capable of ordering longer and longer sequences, so the monitoring demands of movement organization and control become less. The actual length of any sequence, however, is dependent on the environment in which the skill is performed. In closed skills relatively long sequences may be generated and executed since the environment is static and completely predictable. However, in open skills, since the environment is continually changing, the learner can only order a movement that corresponds to a given predictable event. After this he must reanalyze the environment, determine what is necessary in order to achieve his goal, and then generate another sequence of movements to achieve this end.

Gentile (1972), in her model of skill acquisition, calls this second phase of learning the fixation/diversification phase. She uses this term because of the postulated difference underlying the acquisition of open and closed skills. She maintains that in an open skill the learner must diversify his motor schema so that he can generate a unique sequence of movements that match the exact demands of the skill. Since in an open skill no two situations are ever exactly the same, the learner must be able to distinguish the particular characteristics of a given situation and then generate a schema instance to match its demands.

Closed skills, on the other hand, because the environment is static, require that the schema instance become highly fixed or invariable in its execution. Here, the motor schema can be seen as becoming more exact and integrated but for the purpose, unlike that in open skills, of generating the same schema instance time and time again. Also, in closed skills, the learner can build up relatively long sequences of movement since he can predict the exact nature of the environment in advance of execution. Thus, a considerable amount of the learning process would be concerned with establishing long sequences of movement that could be executed without much attention demand.

Considerations in teaching open and closed skills. The fact that open skills must match a constantly varying environment and closed skills are performed in a static environment has implications for the conditions under which these skills should be learned. According to Gentile, as mentioned above, the motor schema of an open skill must be diversified in order that it can meet the demands of any possible environmental situation. The nature of closed skills, on the other hand, appears to require a more fixed schema that is capable of producing the same movement time and time again. Since the theoretical and practical inmplications of this distinction are rather important and of considerable length, a specific section dealing only with this topic will be presented after the present discussion on phases of learning is completed.

Structuring the environment. Given the fact that a learner has developed an idea of the required movement and can perform it relatively well, the next consideration for the instructor is to introduce, in a selective way, environmental cues that the learner has not been required to consider up to this point. It may be, for instance, that in the cognitive phase of learning the instructor simplified the environment so that the total information processing demand was within the capacity of the learner. Now, since some of this information is becoming redundant, and consequently lessening the demand on the information processing system, the instructor can introduce new cues that increase the performance capability of the learner.

In the learning of closed skills this may mean that the instructor gets the learner selectively to attend to cues that, though not drastically influencing performance, do contribute significantly to the achievement of the goal and the execution of the movement. For instance, in many aspects of gymnastics a learner can have a good idea on how to do a stunt, but it may still need refining in terms of the exact position of body parts in relation to the environment in which the movement is being executed. Through instructional sets and augmented feedback the instructor can effectively produce these changes.

In open skills, even though a learner has the approximate spatial/temporal characteristics of the movement mastered, he must still perform the movement in an ever-changing environment. During the first phase of learning the instructor probably would keep the relevant stimuli simple and straightforward, but now they must be made more complicated and thus the practice environment comes more to resemble the actual environment in which the movement will be performed. In essence, this implies that considerable attention must be given to the learning of the perceptual cues that dictate just exactly what the final movement pattern will be. Here, the development of anticipation or prediction ability is very important. This topic was discussed at length in Chapter 4 as part of the perceptual mechanism, and really involves the ability of a performer to predict from environmental cues what the environment will be like at some time in the future. This is necessary because of the time stress under which open skills are usually performed. Without being able to predict future events, a performer would be unable to initiate and execute an appropriate movement in time to meet the exact environmental demand. For example, if a batter were unable to anticipate where a ball, thrown at a speed 100 miles per hour, would cross the plate until it were only a few feet away from him, by the time he initiated and executed his swing the ball would have passed him. The point is, then, that a teacher must give considerable attention to instructing a learner on how to interpret environmental cues that will lead to the ability to predict in advance what will happen.

Having the ability to anticipate environmental events and having the correct movement available for that movement still, however, does not guarantee a successful completion of an open skill. As discussed in Chapter 5 in regard to the decision mechanism, the performer must still be able to match the exact environmental demand with the appropriate movement. Since in any open skill there are very many possible environmental situations and therefore very many variations of the correct movement, a rapid and accurate decision process is of crucial concern. An instructor can facilitate this decision process by teaching for stimulus-response compatibility. This, as described in Chapter 5, is establishing a one-to-one correspondence between a specific environmental demand and its appropriate movement. This ability is obviously developed through performing in a gamelike situation where all possible environmental cues are present and demand all variations of a particular movement. However, it is suggested here that a teacher can facilitate this process in several ways. First, through verbal descriptions the various stimulus-response combinations can be explained to the learner. A second method might be to watch films of a game in slow motion, where the environmental cues can be seen and the appropriate response identified. And third, a teacher can encourage a learner, while resting on the sidelines or watching a game on television, to put himself continually in the position that he would normally assume if he were playing the game. In this way the learner can actually imagine what he would do in particular situations as if he were actually playing the game. He can then evaluate the correctness of his choice of action by observing what occurs during the game he is watching.

The last issue for discussion under this section on structuring the environment during the second phase of learning concerns the introduction of irrelevant or distracting cues in the environment. Up to this point only relevant cues have been mentioned, but certainly in the performance of any skill there will always be irrelevant information in the environment. The noise of crowds is one such source that would apply to the performance of both closed and open skills. In addition, in open skills there are fakes by the opponent, distractions from one's teammates or opponents who are not of central concern at a given time, and perhaps, the distraction of working against time. It is important that performers be able to ignore such environmental information and this, just like the learning of relevant cues, involves a learning process. One can think in terms of the selective attention process discussed in Chapter 4 where, through learning, an individual would assign almost no pertinence to such cues and as a result they would not be selectively attended to. However, this implies that these irrelevant cues must be present in the environment while an individual is learning a movement so that he can learn to ignore them. Thus, the judicious inclusion of these cues by an instructor becomes an important factor during this stage of learning.

Conclusions. During the second phase of learning, a teacher must slowly increase the amount of information presented to the learner. In many cases the exact way this will be done will depend on whether an open or closed skill is being learned. It is important to appreciate, however, that a perceptual-motor skill consists of three component parts (perception, decision and action), and each component has a specific role to play in the successful execution of a movement. Whereas in the first phase of learning the central concern is to establish an idea of the movement and its relevant environmental cues, the second phase is more concerned with introducing cues as they actually occur in gamelike situations. Thus, planning for the introduction of more complex cues that help the performer initiate and control performance become important considerations. Finally, a teacher must give some consideration to the problem of teaching learners how to ignore irrelevant information since this will facilitate their selective attention process.

The Autonomous Phase

The autonomous phase of learning is characterized by performance that becomes increasingly independent of attention demands. Through having learned a skill the performer is able to generate schema instances that exactly match the elements of the skill and, because of redundancy in environmental and proprioceptive cues, the execution of the movement demands very little attention. The attention of the performer can thus be directed to other aspects of performance, such as the overall game strategy. To maintain maximum performance at this phase the performer should definitely not think about the execution of the skill. If attention is brought to bear on these matters, performance will suffer.

One problem that an instructor faces during this final stage of acquisition occurs when an individual's performance, through limitations imposed by the initial structuring of the skill during the previous two phases of learning, limits the performance to a level below his ultimate capacity. For example, a relatively successful golfer, with the advice of a teacher, may decide that the basic swing he uses is not as efficient as it should be, and by changing the swing in certain ways he believes he can ultimately improve his score. To accomplish this, however, the teacher must have the golfer regress back to the associative phase of learning and direct his attention to relevant details of the swing that must be changed. Obviously, when this is done, the new swing will probably not be immediately as efficient as the old swing since the changes will require considerable portions of the central processing capacity and, because of this attention demand, performance will suffer. Nevertheless, through practice the individual should eventually bring the control of the skill back into the autonomous phase and, hopefully, at a higher level of efficiency than the previous one.

One other problem an instructor faces at the autonomous phase of performance is helping to correct the so-called "slump" of highly skilled individuals. Although a slump can be caused by various factors, one obvious source is the unconscious inclusion of errors in information processing somewhere in the chain of mechanisms (perception, decision, and action) that eventually produce the skill. In other words, since the highly skilled individual pays little attention to the initiation and execution of a skill it may be that he eventually starts doing something wrong which leads to unsuccessful performance. Furthermore, since it did happen unconsciously, the performer is unable to pinpoint the problem himself. What he needs is a teacher or coach to analyze the components of the skill systematically, in terms of the perceptual, decision, and action components, to determine where the breakdown in performance is occurring. For example, it may be that a skilled individual comes to analyze the environmental demands of a skill incorrectly because of attending to irrelevant cues. Or it may be that the effector side of performance has been changed significantly from what it originally was, and corrections to the organization of the skill may be needed.

The important point for an instructor to remember in terms of what causes a breakdown in performance is that, as was discussed in Chapters 1 and 2, by watching an individual perform a skill, only one-third of the total process that contributes to a successful performance is apparent—that is, the effector component. To analyze performance in detail the instructor must systematically analyze the other components as well.

The Teaching Model and Open versus Closed Skills

In Chapter 2 considerable space was devoted to contrasting the processes underlying the performance of open and closed skills. Basically, it was pointed out that open skills are those movements performed in an environment where relevant cues are continually changing and successful performance is dependent on how well an individual can match a particular environmental demand with an appropriate movement. As such, as has been emphasized many times in this book, open skills really involve at least three types of learning: perceptual learning, decision learning, and effector learning.

Closed skills, in contrast, are performed in a static environment, where relevant cues do not change during the execution of movement. Thus emphasis in learning is shifted more toward the output or effector side of performance. From this viewpoint, then, a closed skill would seem to be easier to learn than an open skill, since the learner does not have to cope with an ever-changing environment.

Although the above discussion serves to dichotomize open and closed skills at opposite ends of a continuum, in reality there is probably no such thing as a truly closed skill. In fact, the argument to be advanced here, which leads to several teaching implications, is that perhaps there is not as great a difference in these two types of skills as originally indicated. Take, for instance, the requirements for the successful performance of a so-called closed skill, such as pole-vaulting. This skill can actually be thought of as open in nature in that the performer is constantly receiving feedback about his performance. He uses this feedback to monitor his performance and, if the execution of the pole vault at any point in time deviates from some criterion value, the performer must issue the necessary corrections to modify his performance in order for it to be successful. In other words, if one can consider that the pole-vaulter will never be able to replicate an ideal pole vault exactly, performance will tend to vary and as a result the resulting feedback will, just as in an open skill, have to be processed by the perceptual and decision mechanisms in order that some corrective action can be taken. It is important to realize that, because of the speed with which the skill is performed, there will be insufficient time to correct the erroneous part of the movement, but rather a later part will have to be modified to compensate for the poor result of the former part. For instance, in the pole vault, a poor pole placement at takeoff might be able to be compensated for after takeoff by an adjustment of the body position on the pole.

Even if no errors occur in the parts of a closed skill, processes similar to those occurring in open skills will still take place. On some gymnastic stunt where a number of movements are "chained" together, a performer must be able to anticipate not only the sequence of the movements but also their temporal characteristics. Presumably he would do this through learning to anticipate feedback from an early movement so that when it arrives he can use it to cue the initiation of the next movement in the chain of movements. This process would be very similar to a performer's anticipating or predicting environmental cues in an open skill.

The implication of the above examples for teaching is that most closed skills can be considered to have characteristics in common with open skills, where feedback from performing a closed skill can be considered similar to environmental information received while performing an open skill. Implied in this is the fact that teachers should teach closed skills as if they were open in nature. By this is meant that feedback should be considered the same as a variable environmental input that is subject to the limitations of the human information processing system discussed throughout this book. Thus, processes like selective attention, short-term memory, anticipation, and stimulus-response compatibility must all be given consideration by a teacher when instructing individuals who are attempting to learn a closed skill.

The Motor Schema of Open and Closed Skills

At the base of both open and closed skills is the ability to generate a sequence of motor commands (the schema instance) from a generalized source of movement information called the motor schema (see Chapter 7). As indicated in Chapter 7, as well as earlier in the present chapter, it would seem that in an open skill the schema instance would never be the same in repeated performances of a specific skill. This is so because the specific environmental situation with which the movement must be matched will never be the same, and thus the skill will always be required to be performed in somewhat different ways. A closed skill, on the other hand, to be performed ideally, requires a well-structured schema instance that can be generated in the same manner time after time. Undoubtedly, as pointed out in the immediately preceding section of this chapter, there will be some variation from time to time, but the ultimate objective of highly skilled performers would be to produce a schema instance that varied in structure as little as possible on each performance of the skill.

The question of interest now, which has implications for teaching methods, is what learning experiences should an individual be exposed to so that he can develop a motor schema that best suits his needs, whether for an open or a closed skill. Intuitively, it would seem that for an open skill a performer should be exposed to as many environmental situations as possible so that he can attempt to match each situation with an appropriate movement. In essence, this might mean that, after a learner has acquired the basic idea of the skill, he should practice in gamelike situations as much as possible. For it is only in these situations that an individual learns the appropriate types of movements for the many possible different situations.

It follows from this that if a learner is to develop a well-organized and integrated schema of an open skill he must practice in situations that not only will allow the many variations of a movement to be produced but also will require the learner to produce movements that fit the exact environmental demands. For instance, once a learner has the idea of a jump shot in basketball, very little is gained from having him continually practice it without someone checking him. An opponent not only will provide information about when the jump shot should be taken but also will force the learner to modify his shot in subtle ways depending on how the opponent reacts. Learning the jump shot would thus require the development of a diversified schema that was capable of generating a schema instance appropriate to the demands of the environment.

What about the development of a motor schema for a closed skill? In contrast to an open skill, where the motor schema must be capable of generating many variations of the movement, a motor schema for a closed skill must be able to produce very similar movements time after time. From this it would seem that practice of a closed skill should consist of repeated efforts to reproduce the exact correct form of the movement. So if one were attempting to learn a gymnastic stunt, the exact form required would be defined by a teacher, and the learner would attempt to achieve this form through extensive practice.

However, perhaps the development of a motor schema for a closed skill is not as simple as stated above. As mentioned earlier in this chapter, a closed skill can be treated as an open skill if one treats the feedback received from the performance of a closed skill as a source of input to the information processing system. A learner, in the early phases of learning, would have considerable information input (that is, uncertainty) about his performance because of his relative inability to produce a consistent movement. It is proposed here that this feedback is very important for developing the motor schema in that the learner can formulate general rules and principles concerning not only what a correct movement is but also, just as important, what an incorrect movement is. Thus the motor schema is really a generalized structure that is capable of defining the correct parameters of a given movement and has developed through experiencing a wide variety of incorrect and correct movements.

What, in essence, the above view implies is that a motor schema, in order to produce highly structured movements, must have a wide background of movement experiences, the consequences of which have been organized and generalized into principles and rules of movement. Given this type of structure, it matters little whether one is dealing with an open or a closed skill, since the generation of the specific schema instance would involve the same process. The implications of this viewpoint are many. First, it implies that all skilled movement requires a background of general movement knowledge. Second, this knowledge can be transferred to specific movements or skills and facilitate the learning of these skills. And third, once an individual has the idea of a new skill (that is, the cognitive phase of learning, where past experiences have been transferred to the new situation) specific practice in an environment appropriate to where the skill will be performed (for example, during competition) is necessary in order that the motor schema for that particular skill can be fully developed. It is only in this latter aspect of the learning process that open and closed skills would be practiced in different manners.

Since the whole thrust of this section of the present chapter has been to put forward the point of view that open and closed skills are not really as conceptually independent as first indicated, a practical example will be given to illustrate this viewpoint further. This writer has had the good fortune of working at a university where three high jumpers, all capable of jumping more than 7 feet, were working with an excellent coach. Through conversations with the coach and the high jumpers, this writer gained much insight into how a closed skill was learned. The first principle that the coach worked on was that high jumping should be taught as an open skill, where the emphasis is on interpreting feedback as input to the information processing system. In being consistent with this principle, the coach felt it was necessary to develop a background of jumping experiences that would help the high jumpers discriminate and interpret feedback received from high jumping. To operationalize this, the coach would break a season of training (they trained year round) into several periods. For instance, since the ultimate aim of the training program was to have the athletes peak at important competitions, very specific and intense training would occur during the several months preceding this competition. However, during other periods of the year when there was no competition or the competition was relatively unimportant for the overall progression of the athlete, the coach had a more generalized form of training. In particular, he encouraged his athletes to partake in games that demanded jumping into the air and manipulating their bodies while in the air. Sometimes games were invented for this purpose. For example, part of one practice session might be to have the athletes attempt to jump as far as possible and do as many leg and arm movements as possible while in the air. Or, the athletes were sometimes given a basketball and asked to "dunk" the ball in as many different ways as possible. Since they were high jumpers this did not represent a problem, and it was interesting to see the many variations that these athletes came up with.

There were many more types of games given these athletes, but the purpose of having them perform these games was to give them as much experience as possible in handling their bodies in the air. The coach felt that this general jumping experience would benefit the jumper's perception and discrimination of feedback received while high jumping. Although there was no experimental research evidence to indicate whether this was so, it would appear that the principle the coach was working with would be consistent with the view of how the motor schema is developed. In particular, he tried to develop a general motor schema concerned with a generalized source of knowledge about the principles involved in jumping. This schema was developed through each jumper's past experience in jumping and also through the various games played. Then, to develop this schema into a specific form concerned with the skill of high jumping, very specific practice in high jumping was undertaken, at which time the general principles of jumping were used to interpret and discriminate feedback. From this evaluation process, changes in the schema instance were effected, which resulted in better and more efficient ways of high jumping.

It is interesting to note, in the above example, that even though the three athletes were very accomplished high jumpers, the coach, over several years, always included the experience of general jumping activities with the expectation that this would benefit even these highly skilled athletes. In essence, in terms of the theoretical framework established in this book, the coach was actually taking the athletes back to the cognitive phase of learning and attempting to improve their ideas about what was involved in high jumping. By increasing the clarity of the idea or image of the movement, he was hoping ultimately to improve their performance at the autonomous phase of learning.

Implications for Teaching Closed Skills

Development of motor schema. Presumably, except in the very young, every individual comes to a perceptual-motor learning situation with a large amount of past experience relevant to the performance of the new skill. The teacher should develop pertinence for this transfer of information so that the learner can selectively attend to the similarities. Further, even though it is a closed skill, the teacher can supplement this past experience by planning for a wide variety of movement experiences relevant to the learning of a new skill. This experience will presumably help the learner to form rules and principles of movement that will facilitate the acquisition of the to-be-learned skill.

Specificity of practice. Once the learner has the idea of the closed skill, the teacher should plan for practice sessions that develop this general idea into a very specific schema instance that represents the skill itself. This can be accomplished only by practicing under conditions that are as near as possible to the situation that the performer will ultimately have to be tested (compete) in. In keeping with the principle of specificity of practice, the best environment to practice in would be the test or competitive situation itself. However, the fact that an individual is at this phase of learning does not imply that a teacher cannot bring the learner back to the cognitive phase of learning for reasons discussed earlier.

Part-whole versus whole skill practice. Of practical concern when teaching a rather complicated closed skill is the question of whether a skill should be learned in a part-whole manner or by the whole method. For example, when the front crawl in swimming is being taught, in many cases a learner cannot correctly kick his legs, move his arms, and breathe all at the same time. Obviously, the great uncertainty of the feedback (that is, high information load) overloads his information processing system and he is unable to attend to and process all the information at once. Therefore, many teachers, instead of having the learner perform the whole skill rather inadequately, will teach only the kicking action first and then have the learner practice it. Then, when the correct action is achieved, the action of the arms will be introduced separately and then in combination with the legs. Finally, the breathing sequence is taught, at first by itself, and then in combination with the other two components. Some teachers believe that this part-whole method results in faster learning than the use of the whole method.

From the computer analogy of perceptual-motor skills, introduced in Chapter 6, the part-whole method would entail learning each of the subroutines separately and then combining them into a whole, whereas the whole method would require that the total program be practiced. Fitts and Posner (1967, pp. 13–14) provide the best summary of the conflicting research that has attempted to answer the question of which method is best. They state that for most skills, the whole method is superior in that most of the learning is concerned with the integration and timing of the components of the skill. The only time the part-whole method should be utilized is when the skill is so complex that practicing the whole is impossible. However, when this is the case the instructor should break the skill down into component processes that are as nearly independent of each other as possible. Practice should then consist of alternating between part and whole methods.

As an example of the latter principle, when teaching the front crawl in swimming by the part-whole method, an instructor could have a learner practice the leg action by itself since this is relatively independent of the breathing and arm actions. However, the breathing and arm actions should always be practiced together since their sequencing and timing are intrinsically combined. Thus, one way of teaching this skill would be to practice the leg action, then the whole action, then the arm and breathing action, and then the whole action.

Feedback. As mentioned previously in this chapter and in Chapter 7, the successful evaluation of performance is basic to learning. Basically a performer has knowledge of results and performance to evaluate his performance, and this feedback can be augmented by the teacher. Since a closed skill is performed in a relatively static environment, knowledge of results about the outcome of the movement (that is, whether the movement achieved the goal) is relatively unimportant since usually the ultimate concern of a closed skill is how the goal was accomplished. For this reason, emphasis is placed on the performance of the skill, and hence knowledge of performance becomes of crucial concern. The teacher should continuously attempt to aid the learner in selectively attending to feedback concerning the performance of the skill. In addition, most augmented feedback should also be in terms of knowledge of performance.

Implications for Teaching Open Skills

Development of motor schema. For an open skill, as for a closed skill, the development of the motor schema would depend on the existence of already acquired rules and principles of movement. However, in addition to these, the learner would also require some knowledge about the characteristics of relevant cues that control the movement in an open skill. For instance, one prerequisite to catching a ball is that an individual would need to know how to predict ball flight, which means that he has formed rules and principles of the relevant cues on which ball flight is dependent. Thus the motor schema of an open skill would be formed on the basis of both movement and environmental information, and a teacher would have to plan for transfer of information from this already existing knowledge to the learning of the new skill.

Many open skills involve predicting or anticipating ball flight, and an article by Kay (1970) has discussed some of the factors that lead to the anticipation of environmental and proprioceptive cues necessary for catching a ball. He showed that chief among these factors was a developmental trend, probably associated with increasing experience, that explained differences in ball-catching ability among three children, aged 2, 5, and 15 years. From this study it was found that the motor schema for ball catching was fully developed by the age of 15 years but was incomplete at 5 years. Obviously, there would be a wide age range at which such a schema would be developed since it not only would depend on how much experience a learner has in this skill but also would depend on hereditary factors. However, except for children under the age of 5 or 6 years, it might be expected that they would have some past experience in predicting environmental information that the teacher could build upon.

Specificity of practice. Since open skills depend on closely matching environmental situations with relatively exact movements, once the associative phase of learning is reached, a teacher should attempt to keep practices as close as possible to the actual game situation. It is only in this situation that the appropriate pairing of environment and movement can occur. Anything less than a game situation, unless very well planned, has the possibility of introducing artificial situations, and complete transfer to the game situation might not occur. If drills are used, the teacher should carefully consider the environmental-movement relationships in the drill to determine that they are as close to the game situation as possible.

Part-whole versus whole skill learning. While the principle of specificity of practice should, whenever possible, be adhered to, there will be times early in the cognitive or associate phases of learning that performance of the skill in a game situation will be too difficult for an individual. When this is the case, the teacher may have to hold the environment constant while the individual learns the required movement, which, in essence, makes it a closed skill. An example of this might be teaching an overhead clear in badminton by having the learner hit a shuttlecock that is suspended from the ceiling at a height at which it normally would be hit. Here, there is no environmental uncertainty, and therefore the learner can concentrate solely on the performance of the movement. Another example would be a tennis teacher, while instructing the forehand stroke, throwing balls to the learner in such a way that the balls bounced to the same spot every time. Again the environmental uncertainty is reduced so that the individual can acquire the necessary movement before having to use it in a situation where the environment is constantly varying.

If practice, as depicted in the above two examples, can be thought of as roughly equivalent to part-whole learning, where the part is learning a movement in a simplified environment and the whole is learning the movement in a game situation, then the same principle as discussed under closed skills will apply. That is, since open skills involve learning to make sequences of movements to specific environmental demands that vary from moment to moment, practice of these skills should take place in an environment that allows for this type of learning to occur. However, when the skill is too complex to be performed in this manner, the instructor can simplify the environment so that more attention can be given to the performance of the movement. The environment can be simplified in a number of ways: It can be closed, as in the above badminton example; it can be open, but slowed down considerably by having learners move in "slow motion" or by having the ball slowed down (for example, a tennis instructor throwing slow balls to various spots on the court to allow a learner plenty of time to get in position and attempt the correct stroke); or the environment can be simplified by reducing the number of possible alternatives confronting an individual. As an example of this latter point, in a baseball batting practice, the pitcher can be instructed to throw just fast balls so that the batter knows what type of ball will be thrown and can concentrate on learning the appropriate timing involved in hitting such a ball.

Although practice of the above type might at times be necessary, it should be remembered that, in terms of the principle of part-whole practice, the simplified version should always be alternated with the performance of the skill in the "real" situation. And further, there will become a point in learning when the specificity of practice principle should almost always be followed. For instance, once a tennis player has learned to perform a forehand stroke, he should not be encouraged to "groove" this stroke by practicing hitting the ball against a wall. This is totally unrealistic on two counts: first, since tennis is an open skill, no two forehand strokes will ever be performed in the same manner, and therefore a "grooved stroke" is not only unnecessary but will probably hinder performance. And second, because it is an open skill, tennis requires considerable perceptual learning (for example, predicting ball flight, predicting what the opponent will do, and so on), and by hitting a ball against a wall this aspect of learning is completely ignored since most individuals, once they have acquired the stroke, know approximately where the ball will go as it leaves their racket.

Applications of the Information Processing Model to Motor Performance 221

If this type of practice is necessary, a teacher could make the situation a little more realistic by, in the case of the tennis example, having the player practice against an unevenly textured wall, thus making the ball's return somewhat unpredictable.

Feedback. If a teacher simplifies an open skill for a naive learner in order that the movement can be learned without the stress of the real environment in which the skill is normally performed, then the same principle for feedback as discussed under closed skills applies. That is, emphasis should be on the evaluation of the movement, and knowledge of performance is the appropriate type of feedback. Once the learner performs the movement in an open situation however, emphasis is shifted toward whether the outcome of the movement accomplished the goal. In this case, knowledge of results becomes the relevant type of feedback, and a teacher should plan to enhance the process whereby knowledge of results can be used to evaluate performance.

Transfer of Learning

Much of the previous discussion in this chapter has stressed the importance of past experience in the acquisition of a new skill. In fact the concept of the motor schema is based on the premise that a learner has a background of general movement experience that can be used to formulate plans of action for the new skill. Learning from this point of view is seen as applying appropriate past experiences to the requirements of a new skill, and through practice a new motor schema, specific to the new skill, results.

The above concept of learning, then, is heavily dependent on transfer of learning or past experiences. Transfer of learning can be defined as the effect that past experiences have on the learning or performance of a new skill. Although only positive transfer (that is, past experience facilitating the learning of a new skill) has been discussed to this point, in some cases prior experience may have a negative effect on learning a new skill in that the new skill would be interfered with and take longer to learn. An example of where both positive and negative transfer might be expected to occur in a learning situation would be when an individual attempts to learn badminton after he has learned and played tennis. Positive transfer might occur for things like court position action, some aspects of strategy, positioning oneself for stroking, and for some aspects of the stroke itself. Negative transfer might occur when the individual, who is accustomed to the flight characteristics of a tennis ball, tries to switch to the completely different characteristics of a shuttlecock. In addition one might suspect that in stroking the bird, the relatively firm wrist action required for hitting a tennis ball would negatively influence the flexible, whiplike action required for badminton.

Although there are several theories of transfer of learning that attempt to explain why transfer occurs, probably no one theory at the present time is capable of fully describing this complex phenomenon. From the concept of the motor schema described in this book, as well as from the description of the human performance model, where performance is seen to be dependent upon the integration of at least three component parts (perception, decision, and action) one might be able to understand generally what is involved in transfer of learning.

At the base of the motor schema is a generalized source of knowledge concerning the rules and principles of movement. It is built up through years of experience, and even though most individuals are probably incapable of verbally expressing these principles of movement, their actions indicate that they are capable of putting them into operation. These generalized principles of movement probably include information about body control while walking, running, jumping, kicking, and so on, as well as information about the environment and how movements must be matched to the environment to achieve certain goals. For instance, in this latter respect, generalized information about predicting flight characteristics of objects in space, as well as information about movements necessary to intercept these objects with the body, would both be necessary parts of the motor schema. From this viewpoint one would expect that the degree of positive transfer to a new skill would depend on the amount of general past experience an individual has in perceptual-motor skills. The more varied this past experience, the more capable he is in adapting this past experience to a new situation.

Negative transfer probably is caused by a specifically developed motor schema interfering with the formation of another specific schema. For instance, if one learned badminton previous to learning tennis one might expect that the specific perceptual abilities acquired in badminton (for example, learning to predict the flight of the bird) might interfere with the similar perceptual skill of predicting ball flight. Both of these perceptual abilities depend on a common generalized knowledge of flight of objects in space. However, badminton might be expected to interfere with learning tennis because it was a specific concrete outcome of a more generalized source of knowledge, and hence would be the first knowledge a learner might refer to when learning a new skill with similar perceptual demands. Although this example serves to demonstrate how negative transfer might occur due to stimulus or environmental characteristics of a task, the same reasoning can be applied to the response or action phase of performance. Both tennis and badminton rely on swinging a racket, which undoubtedly stems from earlier generalized sources of motor experiences. However, when a specific outcome has been developed (as in stroking a badminton bird), one would expect in learning a new skill requiring a similar action that a learner might use the same specific movement that proved successful in the earlier learned skill. Hence, to the degree that this action is inappropriate to the new skill, negative transfer will occur.

The implications of this view of transfer of learning to the problems of teaching and coaching are numerous, and many suggestions have already been presented in this chapter. Perhaps the most important principle is that a learner should always have new skills expressed in terms of his relevant past experiences. The less the past experience he has, the simpler the level at which the new skill should be introduced. A teacher can facilitate this process by systematically analyzing new skills in terms of their component parts (perceptual, decision, and action) and then attempting to determine how these components have been incorporated in the past movement experiences of the learner.

The fact that the motor schema is based upon a broad generalized source of past movement experiences also has relevance to advocates of the importance of early perceptual-motor experiences in the normal development of a child. While these advocates place considerable emphasis on the importance of perceptual-motor development in the later development of intelligence, the present view would stress that later acquisition of specific perceptual-motor skills is dependent on initially developing a wide base of movement experience. In other words, the development of principles of movement, gained from varied and repeated experiences, would positively transfer to the learning of new skills.

Mental Practice

The emphasis of a good deal of this book has been to treat perceptual-motor skills as cognitive in nature. In other words, theories and evidence have been put forward explaining how perceptual-motor skills are internally represented in the central nervous system and how these representations at times are analogous to images or ideas of movement. An outcome of this is that a plan of action has been discussed as if it were some kind of logical progression of ideas or thoughts that, when grouped together, specify the various parameters of the planned movement. It has been implied, then, that at least for some aspects of perceptual-motor skill performance, there is at least a similarity between the processes underlying this ability and an ability like the logical thinking required to solve intellectual problems. Just as an individual can mentally solve a problem (for example, a logical argument he wants to present) without overtly expressing it, so too can an individual plan a movement in advance and imagine its outcome without actually physically moving.

Although the above is concerned just with movement, part of the plan for action, especially for open skills, must also include knowledge about the relevant environment cues with which the movement must be matched. Learning to recognize and anticipate environment cues can also be considered cognitive in nature in that an individual is capable of representing these events in some form, somewhere in his brain, that allows him to think about them and actually determine the consequences of his thoughts without overtly responding to these cues.

Another aspect of perceptual-motor behavior that is highly cognitive in nature is the establishing of stimulus-response compatibility as defined and discussed in Chapter 5. In essence, this is the process concerned with establishing correspondence between various movements and various environmental demands. One can appreciate that an individual, by watching another individual perform a skill, could come to some conclusion about what responses are associated with specific environmental situations. Thus, this aspect of human performance would also have to be described as cognitive in nature.

The point of the above discussion is an attempt to establish the view that perceptual-motor skills, though their overt manifestations are motor in nature, have a large mental or cognitive component that influences much of the information processing activities concerned with the performance and learning of these skills. In fact, before these skills can be really understood, this writer believes that much more emphasis must be placed on attempting to understand the cognitive nature of these skills. Traditionally, perceptual-motor skills have been treated as pure "motor" in nature with the implication that cognitive abilities played no role in their planning and execution. However, hopefully the previous chapters of this book have established the fact that the only pure motor aspect of a perceptual-motor skill is the actual contraction of muscles, which represents the end point in terms of actually producing movement, but represents only a small part of the total process concerned with organizing, initiating, and controlling that movement.

With this discussion as a framework, the reader might now better appreciate the role that mental practice has in acquiring a perceptual-motor skill. Mental practice can be defined as improvement in performance that results from an individual's either thinking about a skill or watching someone else perform it. To study the effectiveness of mental practice experimentally, usually three groups of subjects are used. All three groups are first tested on the to-be-learned movement; then one group physically practices the skill, the second group either watches someone else perform the skill or just thinks about it, and the third group does nothing. These three groups are then all retested on the skill, and these scores are compared to their original test to see how much improvement took place between test and retest.

When studies have been done using research designs similar to the above, it has been found for a wide variety of perceptual-motor skills that mental practice improves performance over that of individuals who do nothing. In addition, although actual physical practice produces the best improvement, there are indications that judicious combinations of physical and mental practice produce improvements that are just as great.

Although research evidence has not been able to determine exactly why mental practice is effective, the ultimate answer probably lies in the directions suggested at the beginning of this section. That is, to the extent that cognitive abilities underlie the performance and learning of perceptual-motor skills, mental practice will prove beneficial. It is important to realize, however, that different skills, since they change in their reliance on the various underlying component processes, may demonstrate different effects from mental practice. Obviously, what is needed is a skill analysis in terms of the relative contributions of the perceptual, decision, and effector components, and then the determination of what influence mental practice has on skills that vary in reliance on these components. In addition, research is also needed on when, in the various phases of learning, mental practice is most profitable. One would expect, for reasons put forward earlier in this chapter, that the cognitive phase would be most influenced by mental practice, but there is no reason why learning in the other two phases cannot also be facilitated.

Since mental practice obviously influences learning, the teacher should plan to use it in combination with physical practice. Before it can be used effectively, the teacher would be wise to analyze the to-be-learned skill to determine just exactly what components are cognitive in nature and thus probably most influenced by mental practice. Once this is done, mental practice can then be a powerful teaching method. Players sitting on the sidelines can be instructed to watch for certain environmental situations occurring in a game that will help them when they are playing. Similarly, a teacher can direct their attention to stimulus-response relationships important for their performance or, at other times, to the actual physical execution of a movement that might help the observer to obtain a clearer idea or image of the movement.

Generality and Specificity of Perceptual-Motor Skills

In this present chapter there have been two broad principles of perceptual-motor behavior that have been discussed; and, at times, they would seem to contradict each other. One principle concerns how the environment should be structured in order that effective learning can take place. The advice given in this chapter was that a teacher should structure the practice situation to make it exactly resemble the game situation. It was argued that the more realistic a practice was, the more likely the learner would transfer the skill acquired in practice to the real situation in which the skill was to be performed.

The second principle discussed was the broad issue of transfer of learning. In effect, it was pointed out that transfer of learning in situations that sometimes were only generally related to the to-be-learned skill could be expected to occur. In fact, it was argued that a teacher should continually plan, in his instructional methodology, for transfer of learning, especially in the cognitive phase of learning.

The implications of the above two principles, then, would seem to be at first glance contradictory to each other. On the one hand, it is suggested that only very specific practice can be expected to transfer to the real situation; on the other hand, a learner's past general experience is thought to have a great influence on his acquisition of a specific perceptual-motor skill. Are these two viewpoints really contradictory? The view of this writer is that they are not, and the following discussion will be concerned with explaining this viewpoint.

Specificity of Perceptual-Motor Skills

A topic of great interest to individuals concerned with studying perceptual-motor skills has been whether the abilities underlying these skills are general or specific (Marteniuk, 1974). Early investigators had thought that individuals possessed such general abilities as balance, coordination, speed, flexibility, strength, and so on, which determined how well they could learn and perform a large number of specific skills. For instance, those individuals with large amounts of general ability were the so-called all-around athletes, who were good at almost any skill they undertook. On the other hand, those individuals with very little general ability would do poorly at most skills they attempted.

One way of investigating whether general abilities really determined how well an individual performed a specific task was to test a group of individuals on several skills. For example, one might take a group of 30 people and test them on their ability to play badminton, basketball, and tennis. If there was any such thing as general abilities, one might expect that: those individuals with large amounts of ability would perform well on all three tasks; those with medium amounts of ability would perform at a level somewhere in the middle of the group; and those with very little general ability would perform the poorest. On the other hand, if perceptual-motor skills are specific in nature, one would predict that it would just be a matter of chance whether an individual who scored high in one skill would perform high in a second one, or vice versa. In essence, what has to be determined is whether the relative ranking of performance within the group of individuals on a skill like basketball is approximately the same as their ranking on a skill like tennis. If the rankings were the same, some support might be gained for the notion that the two skills were dependent on the same underlying general ability. If the rankings were not the same, and in fact were unrelated, support for the specificity of perceptual-motor skills would be gained.

One way that is commonly used to compare the rankings of a group of individuals on two skills is to compute a correlation coefficient between the scores achieved on one skill with those achieved on the other skill. The resulting correlation coefficient, which can range between -1.0 to $+1.0$, then yields an estimate of the degree to which the individual rankings on the skills are similar. A high positive correlation indicates similar rankings. A low correlation, around zero, indicates that the rankings on one skill are completely unrelated to the rankings on the other skill. Finally, a large negative correlation indicates that the order of ranking on one skill is just the reverse of the ranking on the other skill. Thus, if one suspects that two skills rely on the same underlying ability, it would be predicted that a large positive correlation would result when the two skills were correlated. One word of caution, however, about the interpretation of the correlation coefficient. A high correlation by itself does not imply causality. In other words, a high correlation between two skills may indicate that the scores on the two skills are caused by the same general ability but it could also indicate a relationship for other reasons. For instance, a high correlation could result because of differential motivation among the group of individuals being tested. Those that are highly motivated would perform well on both tests, those that are normally motivated would perform in the middle of the range, and those that were poorly motivated would perform poorly on both tasks. Therefore, before causal relationships can be implied from a correlation coefficient, an investigator must make other logical treatments of his data that preclude the possibility that the correlation is a result of some spurious factor.

When the correlation coefficient has been used to study whether perceptual-motor skills are general or specific, a large amount of evidence (reviewed by Marteniuk, 1974) indicates extreme specificity. Not only does the evidence suggest that performance is specific to a given skill but it also indicates that learning is skill-specific. What this means is that individuals who learn one skill quickly may or may not learn another skill quickly (that is, it is unpredictable). Specificity has also been found in training for such things as strength and speed. In this regard, this means that if one wants to increase his strength in a particular sport, he should devise strength training techniques that utilize the specific movements of the sport. The same principle would apply to training for speed. If one wanted to increase his speed in the 100-yard dash, the best way to do it would be to train specifically in the 100-yard dash rather than working on speed movements that are not found in this skill.

Specificity of Skills and Transfer of Learning

The above discussion would seem to rule out the possibility for transfer of learning to occur. If skills are so highly specific, the only way in which they can be improved would be through specific practice. This would mean that except in those cases where a learner has previously experienced identical elements of the to-be-learned skill (that is, some of the specific environmental cues or movements of the new skill were previously experienced by the learner), one would not expect transfer of learning to occur. However, as discussed previously in this chapter, transfer of learning is seen to have a much broader influence on the acquisition of perceptual-motor skills.

One important reason why the research on specificity of skills and on transfer of learning appear to contradict each other is the interpretation given to the results of those studies concerned with the specificity of skills. As mentioned previously, these studies almost always have used the correlation coefficient as their indicator of specificity, where a low correlation is seen as supporting the concept of specificity. In this respect, a low correlation means that the relative rankings of a group of individuals on one skill is unrelated to their relative rankings on a different skill. However, the fact that this occurs does not preclude the possibility of transfer of learning taking place. The reason for this becomes apparent when one considers the two correlations diagrammed in Figure 34.

Correlation 1 represents the degree to which the relative rankings of six individuals are the same for two tasks, A and B. As can be seen, the relative position of individuals in Task A changes greatly (as indicated by the arrows) when considering their relative performances in Task B. Furthermore, if we can consider that the columns represent standard scores, since the two columns are of equal height and are in the same range of standard scores their means will be exactly the same. Consider now the second correlation, where the only significant change is that the mean performance of one of the tasks (Task D) is much higher than the other task. Since the change in the relative rankings of the six individuals between Tasks C and D is the same as the corresponding change in the first two tasks, the two correlations will be the same. In fact, if one calculates the Spearman Coefficient of Rank Correlation the resulting correlation is

Applications of the Information Processing Model to Motor Performance

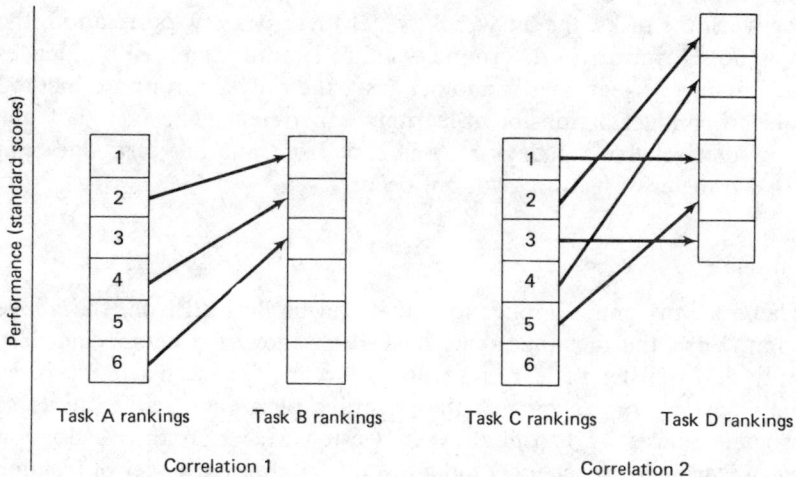

FIGURE 34 The independence of the correlation coefficient and the group mean of performance. See text for how this affects the interpretation of specificity of skills in terms of whether transfer of learning is possible between skills that do not correlate.

0.09. This represents a very low correlation and would be taken as indicating that there was no relationship between Task A and B and between Task C and D.

However, suppose that in correlation 2 in Figure 34 all six individuals had thoroughly learned Task C first and this experience led to the increased mean performance of Task D. This is basically a transfer-of-learning situation where past experience facilitates learning and performance of a new skill. To demonstrate experimentally that transfer took place, another group of individuals, who had not previously learned Task C, would have to be tested on Task D. Their performance on this task should be considerably lower than those who had learned Task C first.

The point is, then, that we have two ways of evaluating whether Tasks C and D have something in common. One is through calculating a correlation between the two tasks, and the other is by determining whether transfer of learning takes place. For the example described, one comes to opposite conclusions depending on whether the correlation is used or the transfer-of-learning design is used. This example serves to point out a serious limitation of the correlation technique; that is, the correlation is insensitive to mean differences between tasks. The correlation is entirely dependent on the relationship between the relative rankings of individuals on two tasks. In other words, it asks the question: If the rank of an individual on one task is known, can the rank of that individual in another task be predicted? If there is a high correlation (either positive or negative in sign) between the tasks, the answer is yes. If there is a low correlation, the answer is no. However, to determine whether learning one task influences the performance or learning of another task, the only appropriate method would be to conduct a transfer-of-learning experiment. The fact that one cannot predict relative rankings on one task from another task does not imply that transfer of learning will not occur.

Implications

There are two main implications that can be derived from the above discussion. First, the fact that skills have been shown to be specific does not imply that transfer of learning will not occur. This seems to have the most implications for teaching at the cognitive phase and earlier parts of the associate phases of learning. As suggested earlier in the section on transfer of learning, a teacher should actively plan to use transfer of training in his methodology. However, in all likelihood, at advanced stages of learning—that is, the late associative phase and autonomous phase—the more specific that practice can be, the more benefits will be derived from it. In this case, the teacher or coach is directly interested in transferring practice behavior to game behavior, and the best way of assuring this transfer is to make the practice situations as gamelike as possible. In this respect, the specificity of performance and learning is a valid concept.

Suggested Readings

The Teaching Model and Phases of Skill Learning

Fitts, P. M., Perceptual-motor skill learning. In Arthur W. Melton (Ed.), *Categories of Human Learning*. New York: Academic Press, 1964.

Gentile, A. M., A working model of skill acquisition with application to teaching. *Quest*, 1972, **17**, 3–23.

Marteniuk, R. G., Information processing, channel capacity, learning stages, and the acquisition of motor skills. In H. T. A. Whiting (Ed.), *Readings in Human Movement*, London: Lepus, 1975a.

Marteniuk, R. G., and Roy, E. A., The codability of kinesthetic location and distance information. *Acta Psychologica*, 1972, **36**, 471–479.

Whiting, H. T. A., *Acquiring Ball Skill, A Psychological Interpretation*, Philadelphia: Lea & Febiger, 1969.

The Teaching Model and Open and Closed Skills

Gentile, A. M., A working model of skill acquisition with application to teaching. *Quest*, 1972, **17**, 3–23.

Marteniuk, R. G., Information processing, channel capacity, learning stages, and the acquisition of motor skills. In H. T. A. Whiting (Ed.), *Readings in Sports Psychology*. London: Henry Kimpton, 1975.

Whiting, H. T. A., *Acquiring Ball Skill, A Psychological Interpretation*. Philadelphia: Lea & Febiger, 1969.

Transfer of Learning

Lindsay, P. H., and Norman, D. A., *Human Information Processing*. New York: Academic Press, 1972.

Singer, R. F., *Motor Learning and Human Performance*. New York: Macmillan, 1968.

Mental Practice

Cratty, B. J., *Movement Behavior and Motor Learning*. Philadelphia: Lea & Febiger, 1973.

Marteniuk, R. G., and Roy, E. A., The codability of kinesthetic location and distance information. *Acta Psychologica*, 1972, **36,** 471–479.

Richardson, A., Mental practice: A review and discussion. *Research Quarterly*, 1967, **38,** 95–107, 263–273.

Generality and Specificity of Perceptual-Motor Skills

Cratty, B. J., *Movement Behavior and Motor Learning*. Philadelphia: Lea & Febiger, 1973.

Marteniuk, R. G., Individual differences in motor performance and learning. In J. A. Wilmore (Ed.), *Exercise and Sport Sciences Reviews*. New York: Academic Press, 1974, 103–130.

Bibliography

Adams, J. A., *Human Memory*. New York: McGraw-Hill, 1967.

Adams, J. A., A closed-loop theory of motor learning. *Journal of Motor Behavior*, 1971, **3,** 111–150.

Adams, J. A., and Dijkstra, S., Short term memory for motor responses. *Journal of Experimental Psychology*, 1966, **71,** 314–318.

Alphern, M., Lawrence, M., and Wolsk, D., *Sensory Processes*. Belmont, Calif.: Brooks/Cole, 1967.

Annett, J., Golby, C. W., and Kay, H., The measurement of elements in an assembly task—the information output of the human motor system. *Quarterly Journal of Experimental Psychology*, 1958, **10,** 1–11.

Attneave, Fred, *Applications of Information Theory to Psychology*. New York: Holt, Rinehart and Winston, 1959.

Attneave, R., and Benson, B., Spatial coding of tactual stimulation. *Journal of Experimental Psychology*, 1969, **81,** 216–222.

Ausubel, D. P., Crucial psychological issues in the objectives, organization and evaluation of curriculum reform movements. *Psychology in the Schools*, 1967, **IV,** 111–121.

Bartlett, F. C., *Remembering: A Study in Experimental and Social Psychology*. New York: Cambridge, 1961.

Berlyne, D. E., *Conflict, Arousal and Curiosity*. New York: McGraw-Hill, 1960.

Bilodeau, E. A. (Ed.), *Principles of Skill Acquisition*. New York: Academic Press, 1969.

Bilodeau, E. A., and Bilodeau, I. McD., Variable frequency of knowledge of results and the learning of a simple skill. *Journal of Experimental Psychology*, 1958a, **55,** 379–383.

Bilodeau, E. A., and Bilodeau, I. McD., Variation of temporal intervals among critical events in five studies of knowledge of results. *Journal of Experimental Psychology*, 1958b, **55,** 603–612.

Bilodeau, E. A., Bilodeau, I. McD., and Schumsky, D. A., Some effects of introducing and withdrawing knowledge of results early and late in practice. *Journal of Experimental Psychology*, 1959, **58,** 142–144.

Bilodeau, E. A., Sulzer, J. L., and Levy, C. M., Theory and data on the inter-relationships of three factors of memory. *Psychological Monograph*, 1962, **76,** (No. 539), 20.

Bilodeau, I. McD., Accuracy of a simple positioning response with variation in the number of trials by which knowledge of results is delayed. *American Journal of Psychology*, 1956, **69,** 434–437.

Birch, H. G., and Lefford, A., Visual differentiation, intersensory integration, and voluntary motor control. *Monographs of the Society for Research in Child Development. Serial #110*, 1967, **32,** No. 2.

Birch, D., and Veroff, J., *Motivation: A Study of Action*. Belmont, Calif.: Brooks/Cole, 1966.

Brindley, G. S., and Merton, P. A., The absence of position sense in the human eye. *Journal of Physiology*, 1960, 153, 127–130.

Broadbent, D. E., *Perception and Communication*. London: Pergamon Press, 1958.

Cardozo, B. L., and Leopold, F. F., Human code transmission: letters and digits compared on the basis of immediate memory error rates. *Ergonomics*, 1963, **6,** 133–141.

Celli, Barbara, and Rothstein, Anne, Applications of the learning model: basketball foul shot. *Bridging the Gap*, 1972, **2,** Nos. 1 & 2.

Chase, R. A., An information-flow model of the organization of motor activity. Part I: Transduction, transmission, and central control of sensory information. *Journal of Nervous and Mental Disease*, 1965a, **140,** 239–251.

Chase, R. A., An information-flow model of the organization of motor activity. Part II: Sampling, central processing, and utilization of sensory information. *Journal of Nervous and Mental Disease*, 1965b, **140,** 334–350.

Chernikoff, R., and Taylor, F. V., Reaction time to kinesthetic stimulation resulting from sudden arm displacement. *Journal of Experimental Psychology*, 1952, **43,** 1–8.

Cherry, E. C., Some experiments on the recognition of speech, with one and two ears. *Journal of the Acoustical Society of America*, 1953, **25,** 975–979.

Cleghorn, T. E., and Darcus, H. D., The sensibility to passive movement of the human elbow joint. *Quarterly Journal of Experimental Psychology*, 1952, **4,** 66–79.

Cofer, C. N., and Appley, M. H., *Motivation: Theory and Research*. New York: Wiley, 1964.

Connolly, K. (Ed.), *Mechanisms of Motor Skill Development*. New York: Academic Press, 1970.

Connolly, K., and Jones, B., A developmental study of efferent-reafferent integration. *British Journal of Psychology*, 1970, **61,** 259–266.

Cratty, B. J., *Movement Behavior and Motor Learning*. Philadelphia: Lea & Febiger, 1973.

Crossman, E. R. F. W., The measurement of discriminability. *Quarterly Journal of Experimental Psychology*, 1955, **7,** 176–195.

Crossman, E. R. F. W., Information processes in human skill. *British Medical Bulletin*, 1964, **20,** 32–37.

Crossman, E. R. F. W., and Goodeve, P. J., *Feedback Control of Hand-Movement and Fitts' Law.* Communication to the Experimental Psychology Society, 1963.

Davey, C. P., Physical exertion and mental performance. *Ergonomics*, 1973, **16,** No. 5, 595–599.

Davies, B. T., Sensitivity of joint rotation. *Ergonomics*, 1966, **9,** 217–324.

Duffy, E., *Activation and Behavior.* New York: Wiley, 1962.

Duffy, E., The concept of activation. In R. N. Haber (Ed.), *Current Research in Motivation.* New York: Holt, Rinehart and Winston, 1968.

Eldred, E., Peripheral receptors: their excitation and relation to reflex patterns. *American Journal of Medicine*, 1967, **46,** 69–87.

Eriksen, C. W., and Johnson, H. J., Storage and decay characteristics of nonattended auditory stimuli. *Journal of Experimental Psychology*, 1964, **8,** 28–36.

Eysenck, J., *The Biological Basis of Personality.* Springfield, Ill.: Charles C Thomas, 1967.

Fiske, D. W., and Maddi, S. R., *Functions of Varied Experience.* Homewood, Ill.: Dorsey Press, 1961.

Fitts, P. M., The information capacity of the human motor system in controlling the amplitude of movement. *Journal of Experimental Psychology*, 1954, **47,** 381–391.

Fitts, P. M., Perceptual-motor skill learning. In Arthur W. Melton (Ed.), *Categories of Human Learning.* New York: Academic Press, 1964.

Fitts, P. M., and Peterson, J. R., Information capacity of discrete motor responses. *Journal of Experimental Psychology*, 1964, **67,** 103–112.

Fitts, P. M., and Posner, M. I., *Human Performance.* Belmont, Calif.: Brooks/Cole, 1967.

Fleishman, E. A., and Rich, S., Role of kinesthetic and spatial-visual abilities in perceptual motor learning. *Journal of Experimental Psychology*, 1963, **66,** 6–11.

Gagné, R. M., *The Conditions of Learning.* New York: Holt, Rinehart and Winston, 1965.

Garner, W. R., An informational analysis of absolute judgments of loudness. *Journal of Experimental Psychology*, 1953, **46,** 373–380.

Garner, W. R., and Hake, H. W., Amount of information in absolute judgments. *Psychological Review*, 1951, **58,** 446–459.

Gentile, A. M., A working model of skill acquisition with application to teaching. *Quest*, 1972, **17,** 3–23.

Goldscheider, A., Unterduchungen über den Muskelsinn. *Archives of Anatomy and Physiology*, 1889, 392–502.
Goodwin, G. M., McCloskey, D. I., and Matthews, P. B. C., Proprioceptive illusions induced by muscle vibration: contribution by muscle spindles to perception. *Science*, 1972, **175,** 1382–1384.
Gottsdanker, R., and Stelmach, G. E., The persistence of psychological refractoriness. *Journal of Motor Behavior*, 1971, **3,** 301–312.
Granit, Ragnar, Constant errors in the execution and appreciation of movement. *Brain*, 1972, **95,** 649–660.
Green, D. M., and Swets, J. A., *Signal Detection Theory and Psychophysics.* New York: Wiley, 1966.
Haber, R. H., Introduction to *Information Processing Approaches to Visual Perception.* New York: Holt, Rinehart and Winston, 1969.
Hebb, D. O., *The Organization of Behavior.* New York: Wiley, 1949.
Hebb, D. O., Drives and the C.N.S. (conceptual nervous system), *Psychological Review*, 1955, **62,** 243–254.
Henmon, V. A. C., The time of perception as a measure of differences in sensation. *Archives of Philosophical and Psychological Scientific Methods*, 1906, No. 8.
Holding, D. H., *Principles of Training.* New York: Pergamon, 1965.
Houk, James, and Henneman, Elwood, Feedback control of movement and posture. *Medical Physiology*, 1967, 1681–1696.
Howard, I. P., and Templeton, W. B., *Human Spatial Orientation.* New York: Wiley, 1966.
Hyman, R., Stimulus information as a determinant of reaction time. *Journal of Experimental Psychology*, 1953, **45,** 188–196.
Jones, B., and Connolly, L., Memory effects in cross-model matching. *British Journal of Psychology*, 1970, **61,** 267–270.
Kahneman, D., *Attention and Effort.* Englewood Cliffs, N.J.: Prentice-Hall, 1973.
Kay, H., Channel capacity and skilled performance. In F. A. Geldard (Ed.), *Defence Psychology.* New York: Macmillan, 1962.
Kay, H., Analyzing motor skill performance. In K. Connolly (Ed.), *Mechanisms of Motor Skill Development.* New York: Academic Press, 1970.
Keele, S. W., Movement control in skilled motor performance. *Psychological Bulletin*, 1968, **70,** 387–403.
Keele, S. W., *Attention and Human Performance.* Pacific Palisades, Calif.: Goodyear, 1973.
Keele, S. W., and Ells, J. G., Memory characteristics of kinesthetic information. *Journal of Motor Behavior*, 1972, **4,** 127–134.
Keele, S. W., and Posner, M. I., Processing of visual feedback in rapid movement. *Journal of Experimental Psychology*, 1968, **77,** 155–158.

Kerr, B., Processing demands during mental operations. *Memory and Cognition*, 1973, **1,** 401–412.

Klemmer, E. T., Simple reaction time as a function of time uncertainty. *Journal of Experimental Psychology*, 1957, **54,** 195–200.

Konorski, J., *Integrative Activity of the Brain*. Chicago: University of Chicago Press, 1967.

Koster, W. G. (Ed.), *Attention and Performance II*. Amsterdam: North-Holland, 1969.

Laabs, Gerald J., Retention characteristics of different reproduction cues in motor short-term memory. *Journal of Experimental Psychology*, 1973, **100,** 168–177.

Lashley, K. S., The problem of serial order in behavior. In L. A. Jeffress (Ed.), *Cerebral Mechanisms in Behavior: The Nixon Symposium*. New York: Wiley, 1951.

Laszlo, Judith I., and Bairstow, P. J., Accuracy of movement, peripheral feedback and efference copy. *Journal of Motor Behavior*, 1971, **3,** 241–252.

Lavery, J. J., and Suddon, Florence H., Retention of simple motor skills as a function of the number of trials by which KR is delayed. *Perceptual Motor Skills*, 1962, **15,** 231–237.

Lembo, John M., *The Psychology of Effective Classroom Instruction*. Columbus, Ohio: Merrill, 1969.

Leonard, J. A., Tactual choice reactions. *Quarterly Journal of Experimental Psychology*, 1959, **11,** 76–83.

Lindsay, P. H., and Norman, D. A., *Human Information Processing*. New York: Academic Press, 1972.

Lindsley, D. B., Emotion. In S. S. Stevens (Ed.), *Handbook of Experimental Psychology*. New York: Wiley, 1951, 473–516.

Mackworth, J. F., The duration of the visual image. *Canadian Journal of Psychology*, 1963, **71,** 62–81.

Malmo, R. B., Activation: a neuropsychological dimension. *Psychological Review*, 1959, **66,** 367–386.

Marteniuk, R. G., Motor performance and induced muscular tension. *Research Quarterly*, 1968, **39,** 4.

Marteniuk, R. G., An informational analysis of active kinesthesis as measured by amplitude of movement. *Journal of Motor Behavior*, 1971, **3,** 1.

Marteniuk, R. G., Retention characteristics of motor short-term memory. *Journal of Motor Behavior*, 1973, **5,** 249–259.

Marteniuk, R. G., Individual differences in motor performance and learning. In J. A. Wilmore (Ed.), *Exercise and Sport Sciences Reviews*. New York, Academic Press, 1974, 103–130.

Marteniuk, R. G., Information processing, channel capacity, learning stages, and the acquisition of motor skills. In H. T. A. Whiting (Ed.), *Readings in Human Movement*. London: Lepus, 1975a.

Marteniuk, R. G., Information processing in motor short-term memory and in the execution of movement. In H. T. A. Whiting (Ed.), *Readings in Human Movement*. London: Lepus, 1975b.

Marteniuk, R. G., and Hayes, K., Kinesthetic information and the control of movement. In H. T. A. Whiting (Ed.), *Readings in Human Movement*. London: Lepus, 1975.

Marteniuk, R. G., and Roy, E. A., The codability of kinesthetic location and distance information. *Acta Psychologica*, 1972, **36,** 471–479.

Marteniuk, R. G., Shields, H., and Campbell, S., Amplitude, position, timing and velocity as cues in reproduction of movement. *Perceptual and Motor Skills*, 1972, **35,** 51–58.

Martens, R., Arousal and motor performance. In J. A. Wilmore (Ed.), *Exercise and Sport Sciences Reviews*. New York: Academic Press, 1974.

McNicol, D., *A Primer of Signal Detection Theory*. London: G. Allen, 1972.

Melton, A. W., Implications of short-term memory for a general theory of memory. *Journal of Verbal Learning and Verbal Behavior*, 1963, **2,** 1–21.

Merton, P. A., Absence of conscious position sense in the human eyes. In M. B. Bender (Ed.), *The Oculomotor System*. New York: Harper & Row, 1964.

Miller, G. A., The magical number seven plus or minus two: some limits on our capacity for processing information. *Psychological Review*, 1956, **63,** 81–97.

Miller, G. A., Galanter, E., and Pribram, K. H., *Plans and the Structure of Behavior*. New York: Holt, Rinehart and Winston, 1960.

Milner, B., The memory defect in bilateral hippocampal lesions. *Psychiatric Research Reports*, 1959, **11,** 43–52.

Moray, N., *Listening and Attention*. London: Penguin Press, 1970.

Mountcastle, V. B. and Powell, T. P. S., Central nervous mechanisms subserving position sense and kinesthesis. *Bulletin of the Johns Hopkins Hospital*, 1959, **105,** 173–200.

Mowbry, G. H., Choice reaction times for skilled responses. *Quarterly Journal of Experimental Psychology*, 1960, **12,** 193–202.

Mowbry, G. H., and Rhoades, M. V., On the reduction of choice reaction times with practice. *Quarterly Journal of Experimental Psychology*, 1959, **11,** 16–23.

Nacson, J., Organization of practice and acquisition of a simple motor task. Presented at the First Canadian Congress for the Multi-Disciplinary Study of Sport and Physical Activity, October, 1973.

Nacson, J., Jaeger, M., and Gentile, A., Encoding processes in short-term motor memory. *Proceedings of the Fourth Canadian Psycho-motor Learning and Sport Psychology Symposium*, University of Waterloo, Waterloo, Canada, 1972.

Neisser, V., *Cognitive Psychology*. New York: Appleton-Century-Crofts, 1967.

Norman, D. A., *Memory and Attention*. New York: Wiley, 1969.

Peterson, L. R., and Peterson, M., Short-term retention of individual items. *Journal of Experimental Psychology*, 1959, **58,** 193–198.

Pew, R. W., Acquisition of hierarchical control over the temporal organization of a skill. *Journal of Experimental Psychology*, 1966, **71,** 764–771.

Pew, R. W., Levels of analysis in motor control. *Brain Research*, 1974, **71,** 393–400.

Pew, R. W., Human perceptual-motor performance. In B. H. Kantowitz (Ed.), *Human Information Processing: Tutorials in Performance and Cognition*. Hillsdale, N.J.: Erlbaum, 1974.

Pillsbury, W. B., Does the sensation of movement originate in the joint? *American Journal of Psychology*, 1901, **XXII,** 346–353.

Pollack, I., The information of elementary auditory displays, I. *Journal of the Acoustical Society of America*, 1952, **24,** 745–749.

Posner, M. I., Characteristics of visual and kinesthetic memory codes. *Journal of Experimental Psychology*, 1967, **74,** 103–107.

Posner, M. I., Short term memory systems in human information processing. In R. N. Haber (Ed.), *Information-Processing Approaches to Visual Perceptions*. New York: Holt, Rinehart and Winston, 1969.

Posner, M. I., and Boies, S. J., Components of attention. *Psychological Review*, 1971, **78,** 391–408.

Posner, M. I. and Keele, S. W., Attention demands of movements. *Proceedings of the Sixteenth International Congress of Applied Psychology*. Amsterdam: Swets and Zeitlinger, 1969.

Posner, M. I., and Keele, S. W., Time and space as measures of mental operations. *Proceedings of the 78th Annual Convention of the American Psychological Association*, 1970.

Posner, M. I., and Keele, S. W., Skill learning. In R. M. W. Travers (Ed.), *Handbook of Research on Teaching*. Washington, D.C.: American Educational Research Association, 1972.

Posner, M. I., and Konick, A. F., Short-term retention of visual and kinesthetic information. *Organizational Behavior and Human Performance*, 1966, **1,** 71–86.

Poulton, E. C., On prediction in skilled movement. *Psychological Bulletin*, 1957, **54,** 467–478.

Reynolds, D., Time and event uncertainty in unisensory reaction time. *Journal of Experimental Psychology*, 1966, **71,** 286–293.

Richardson, A., Mental practice: A review and discussion. *Research Quarterly*, 1967, **38**, 95–107, 263–273.

Rothkopf, E. Z., Some theoretical and experimental approaches to problems in written instruction. In *Learning and the Educational Process*. Skokie, Ill.: Rand McNally, 1965.

Rothstein, Anne, Facilitation of learning through the application of the TOTE model. *Bridging the Gap*, 1972, **2**, Nos. 4 & 5.

Russell, D. G., and Marteniuk, R. G., An information analysis of absolute judgments of torque. *Perception and Psychophysics*, 1974, **16**, 443–448.

Schmidt, R. A., Anticipation and timing in human motor performance. *Psychological Bulletin*, 1968, **70**, 631–646.

Schmidt, R. A., *Motor Skills*. New York: Harper & Row, 1975.

Schmidt, R. A., A schema theory of discrete motor skill learning, *Psychological Review*, 1975, **82**, 225–260.

Schutz, R. W., and Roy, E. A., Absolute error: the devil in disguise. *Journal of Motor Behavior*, 1973, **5**, 141–155.

Scott, M. G., *Analysis of Human Motion*. New York: Appleton, 1945.

Scott, W. E., Jr., Activation theory and task design. *Organizational Behavior and Human Performance*, 1966, **1**, 3–30.

Singer, R. F., *Motor Learning and Human Performance*. New York: Macmillan, 1968.

Smith, Judith L., Kinesthesis: A model for movement feedback. In R. C. Brown and B. J. Cratty (Eds.), *New Perspectives of Man in Action*, Englewood Cliffs, N.J.: Prentice-Hall, 1969.

Smith, Marilyn, Theories of the psychological refractory period. *Psychological Bulletin*, 1967, **67**, 202–213.

Sperling, G., The information available in brief visual presentations. *Psychological Monographs*, 1960, 74.

Stelmach, G. E., Retention of motor skills. In J. A. Wilmore (Ed.), *Exercise and Sport Sciences Review*. New York: Academic Press, 1974.

Stelmach, G. E., and Bassin, S. L., The role of overt motor rehearsal in kinesthetic recall. *Acta Psychologica*, 1971, **35**, 56–63.

Swets, J. A., Indices of signal detectability obtained with various psychophysical procedures. *Journal of the Acoustical Society of America*, 1959, **31**, 511–513.

Swets, J. A., *Signal Detection and Recognition by Human Observers*. New York: Wiley, 1964.

Swets, J. A., Tanner, W. P., and Birdsall, T. G., Decision processes in perception. *Psychological Review*, 1961, **68**, 301–340.

Tanner, W. P., and Swets, J. A., A decision-making theory of visual detection, *Psychological Review*, 1954, **61**, 401–409.

Taub, E., and Berman, A. J., Movement and learning in the absence of sensory feedback. In S. J. Freedman (Ed.), *The Neuropsychology of Spatially Oriented Behavior*. Homewood, Ill.: Dorsey Press, 1968.

Treisman, A. M., Monitoring and storage of irrelevant messages in selective attention. *Journal of Verbal Learning and Verbal Behavior*, 1964, **3**, 449–459.

Trowbridge, M. H., and Cason, H., An experimental study of Thorndike's theory of learning. *Journal of General Psychology*, 1932, **7**, 245–258.

Vince, M. A., Corrective movements in a pursuit task. *Quarterly Journal of Experimental Psychology*, 1948, **1**, 85–103.

Vince, M. A., Rapid response sequences and the psychological refractory period. *British Journal of Psychology*, 1949, **40**, 23–40.

Von Holst, E., Relations between the central nervous system and the peripheral organs. *British Journal of Animal Behavior*, 1954, **II**, 89–94.

Weinberg, D. R., Guy, D. E., and Tupper, R. W., Variations of postfeedback interval in simple motor learning, *Journal of Experimental Psychology*, 1964, **67**, 98–99.

Welford, A. T., Aging and Human Skill. New York: Oxford, 1958.

Welford, A. T., The measurement of sensory-motor performance: survey and reappraisal of twelve years progress. *Ergonomics*, 1960, **3**, 189–230.

Welford, A. T., *Fundamentals of Skill*. London: Methuen, 1968.

Welford, A. T., Stress and performance. *Ergonomics*, 1973, **16**, 567–580.

Whiting, H. T. A., *Acquiring Ball Skill, A Psychological Interpretation*. Philadelphia: Lea & Febiger, 1969.

Wilberg, Robert B., and Salmela, John H., Information load and response consistency in sequential short-term motor memory. *Perceptual and Motor Skills*, 1973, **37**, 23–29.

Williams, Harriet G., Neurological concepts and perceptual-motor behavior. In R. C. Brown, Jr. and B. J. Cratty (Eds.), *New Perspectives of Man in Action*. Englewood Cliffs, N.J.: Prentice-Hall, 1969.

Winter, J. E., The sensation of movement. *Psychological Review*, 1912, **19**, 374–385.

Woodworth, R. S., and Schlosberg, H., *Experimental Psychology*. New York: Holt, Rinehart and Winston, 1954.

Yerkes, R. M., and Dodson, J. D., The relation of strength of stimulus to rapidity of habit formation. *Journal of Comparative Neurology and Psychology*, 1908, **18**.

Index

Absolute judgment, 64–67
  and tennis, 21
  and kinesthesis, 72–75
Activation, determinants of, 42–44
Activation theory, 40–42
  and individual differences, 44
  and signal detection theory, 53–61
Adams, J. A., 9, 73, 182, 206
Adams, J. A. and Dijkstra, S., 93, 163
Alertness (*see* Activation and Attention)
Anticipation, 98–102
  of feedback, 141–152
  hitting and catching a ball, 99
  proprioceptive feedback, 100
  reaction time, 98
  selective attention, 98
  in tennis, 21–22
  timing of movements, 101–102
Attention, 195–196
  as alertness, 39–46
  and limited information processing concept, 46–48
  and movement control, 135
  and space, 46
  See also Information processing
  See also Selective attention
Attneave, F. and Benson, B., 175
Augmented knowledge of performance, 178
Augmented knowledge of results, 178
Ausubel, D. P., 147

Bartlett, F. C., 168
Bilodeau, I., 183
Bilodeau, E. A. and Bilodeau, I., 182
Bilodeau, E. A., Bilodeau, I., and Schumsky, D. A., 181
Bilodeau, E. A., Sulzer, J. L., and Levy, C. M., 163
Birch, D. and Lefford, A., 171
Birch, D. and Veroff, J., 41
Broadbent, D. E., 78

Cardozo, B. L. and Leopold, F. F., 87
Chernikoff, R. and Taylor, F. V., 133
Cherry, E. C., 77
Choice reaction time (*see* Decision mechanism)
Cleghorn, T. E. and Darcus, H. D., 70
Closed-loop control, 139
  See also Movement control
Closed-loop theory of motor learning, 73
Closed skills, 15, 27–28
Coding of information, 9, 14, 161, 197
Complexity, 47
Connolly, K. and Jones, B., 171
Crossman, E. R. F. W., 6, 50
Crossman, E. R. F. W. and Goodeve, P. J., 133

Davey, C. P., 43
Davies, B. T., 70
Decision mechanism, 6, 106–127
  and event uncertainty (choice reaction time), 112
  and golf, 28
  and perceptual discrimination, 115
  and reaction time, 106–107, 111–123
  and teaching, 33
  and temporal uncertainty, 111
  and tennis, 23–24
Detection, 51–61
  of kinesthetic information, 69–70
Difference threshold (*see* Information comparison)
Difficulty, Index of, 130, 131
  (*See also* Fitts' law)
Duffy, E., 41

Effector mechanism, 128–151
  and golf, 28
  and teaching, 33
  and tennis, 25–27
Efference, 14
Eldred, E., 68

Eriksen, C. W. and Johnson, H. J., 9
Eysenck, J., 44

Feedback, 13, 177–184, 218, 221
  anticipation of, 140–141
  index of difficulty, 131
  learning and Fitts' law, 134
  proprioceptive and kinesthetic, 13–14
  time to process, 132, 133
  See also Knowledge of results
Fiske, D. W. and Maddi, S. R., 42
Fitts, P. M., 129, 131, 205, 206
Fitts' law, 130, 137
Fitts, P. M. and Peterson, J. R., 130
Fitts, P. M. and Posner, M. I., 62, 85, 88, 117, 121, 145, 205, 218
Fleishman, E. A. and Rich, S., 204

Gagné, R. M., 147
Generality vs. specificity, 225–230
Gentile, A. M., 75, 178, 207
Goldschneider, A., 70
Goodwin, G. M., McCloskey, D. I., and Matthews, P. B. C., 68
Gottsdanker, R. and Stelmach, G. E., 122

Haber, R. H., 156
Hebb, D. O., 169
Helmholtz, H., 107
Henmon, V. A. C., 115
Hierarchical and sequential organization
  and golf, 28
  and movement control, 144–151
  and tennis, 25–26
  See also Movement control
Houk, J. and Henneman, E., 69
Howard, I. P. and Templeton, W. B., 68
Human performance theory, 5
  "black-box" approach, 6
  limiting principle, 7
Hyman, R., 114

Information, 12
Information comparison, 61–67

Information measurement, 108–111
  index of movement difficulty, 130, 131
Information processing, 12
  and inverted-U hypothesis, 45–46
  and learning, 125
  time and attention as limiting factors, 123–126
Information transmission, 12
Intersensory integration, 170–177
Inverted-U hypothesis, 40
  and information processing, 45–46

Jones, B. and Connolly, K., 171
Just noticeable difference (*see* Information comparison)

Kahneman, D., 39
Kay, H., 83, 131
Keele, S. W., 9, 10, 14, 46, 68, 85, 88, 117, 122, 123, 125, 130, 133, 137, 156, 161, 162
Keele, S. W. and Ells, J. G., 92
Keele, S. W. and Posner, M. I., 132
Kinesthesis, 67–74
  See also Short-term memory
Klemmer, E. T., 111
Knowledge of performance, 14, 177–184, 201
Knowledge of results, 14, 177–184, 201
Konorski, J., 171

Laabs, G. J., 92, 94
Lashley, K. S., 170, 175
Laszlo, J. I. and Bairstow, P. J., 157
Lavery, J. J. and Suddon, F. H., 183
Learning, 155–185
  capacity of effector mechanisms, 130
  Fitts' law and feedback, 134
  knowledge of performance, 177
  knowledge of results, 177
  model, 173
  part-whole vs. whole methods, 217, 219
  and short-term memory, 160–168
  transfer of, 221–223
Learning phases, 203–212